NARCOTIC PLANTS

Revised and Enlarged

*Other books
by the same author*

BIZARRE PLANTS

SARAH BERNHARDT

NARCOTIC PLANTS

Revised and Enlarged

WILLIAM EMBODEN

MACMILLAN PUBLISHING CO., INC.

NEW YORK

Macmillan Publishing Co., Inc.
866 Third Avenue, New York, N.Y. 10022
Collier Macmillan Canada, Ltd.

Library of Congress Cataloging in Publication Data
Emboden, William A
  Narcotic plants
  Bibliography: p.
  1. Psychotropic plants. I. Title.
QK99.A1E5 1979   581.6'34   79–11758
ISBN –02–535480–9

Designed by Philip Grushkin

First Printing 1979

Printed in the United States of America

Dedicated to the memory of
"Rocky" (1970–1977)

"Who possessed beauty without vanity,
Strength without insolence,
Courage without ferocity,
And all the virtues of man without his vices."

Lord Byron's Epitaph for
"Boatswain" 1808

CONTENTS

PREFACE

In 1972, Macmillan Publishing Company, Inc., New York, and Studio Vista, London, jointly published my book *Narcotic Plants*. This volume became something of a landmark in that it presented the botany of psychoactive plants of the world, with many illustrations in color for the first time, and presented the reader with a comprehensive appendix indicating the chemical principle present, the geographical distribution, and some salient botanical features. It has now become evident that a rewrite of that first edition with much new information is long overdue. The discipline of ethnobotany has made rapid strides in less than a decade, and there is more information available as well as greater accuracy concerning the chemical composition of these plants, tolerable levels in the human body, and the context of use in diverse parts of the world.

As with the original volume *Narcotic Plants*, the author will reserve judgement with respect to the mores involved in the use of these plants or their products. Societal judgements are changing rapidly as misconceptions about psychoactive plants are being dispelled. Subcultures centered on the use of one or more drug plants are common throughout the world, and it is the task of sociologist, psychologist, and political figures to make decisions concerning states of drug intoxication. The ethnobotanist should reserve his personal judgement in an exposition such as this, for it can be little more than sorting through the plethora of controversy and selecting those arguments that to him seem most compelling. Thus, the author must refrain from becoming the advocate of either the drug cultures or those who are attempting to annihilate such groups. A dispassionate observer is likely to eventually gain a better perspective on drug use in both a historical and a contemporaneous setting than one who rushes into judgements.

The phenomenon of using psychoactive plants that many thought to be the trivial passing madness of the 1960's is more alive today in civilized areas of the world than it was in that decade. The numbers of journals and magazines devoted to the drug culture increase yearly. In those publications that cater to the user, the number of plant drugs has increased, their mode of cultivation has been widely promulgated, bizarre methods of usage are explained, and the "high priests" of these cults speak out with seeming impunity. The organization of at least one church devoted to psychoactive sacraments has taken place in recent years, and publications emanating from this religious organization enumerate the ever-increasing species of psychoactive plants that constitute their sacraments.

Another kind of publication becoming popular in major cities is the drug analysis sheet giving the reader insights into the drugs being marketed, the names under which they are sold, and an analysis from a competent laboratory. An overview of the results of one such publication, *Pharmchem Survey*, indicates that a number of street drugs of alleged plant origin are misrepresented to the gullible purchaser.

The response from law enforcement agencies has been diverse. We have seen the penalties associated with the use of *Cannabis* evolve to the harshness of a fine associated with a parking ticket in major cities. The attempt to find and exterminate the centers of origin of plant drugs has been stepped up and the penalties are of ominous severity. More sophisticated instrumentation is now being used by law enforcement agencies in many areas. Unfortunately, many still resort to simplistic, non-specific, screening techniques in futile attempts to "identify" alleged narcotic plant materials. Courts in most cities spend a disproportionate amount of time attempting to sort out the rights and wrongs of this behavioral pattern as though court decisions conditioned behavior. Evidence is to the contrary.

Many schools from junior high schools to universities are actively involved in "drug abuse" courses. The trend is now toward an analysis of the possible physical and legal consequences of such behavior. More sophisticated schools have active programs of ethnobotanical surveys that put these plants into a historical and cultural perspective, avoiding the blanket condemnations that cause students to turn a deaf ear.

We are a drug culture: from the first cup of coffee and the cigarette in the morning, through the martini before dinner, into the wines and aperitifs, and finally the tranquilizer that, despite warnings to the contrary, is popped before bedtime. The question now seems to be to what degree will a drug culture tolerate a drug subculture whose drug choices are different? We may view with horror, or become informed as to the nature of these patterns of behavior different from our own. The view from the castle can only create a greater alienation within families and between age groups than already exists. It seems imperative, therefore, that we all become informed with regard to each other's respective poisons and passions before making critical judgements. This book is an attempt to present data on drug plants in historical perspective with the absence of hysteria, condemnation, or approbation. Prohibitions against Egyptians had as little effect as the prohibitions of today. Such uninformed propaganda as the film *Reefer Madness* is now viewed as a comedy flick to be seen on late night television.

The latest innovation among drug subcultures seems to be the ascendancy of plant drugs among the affluent white community that was formerly thought to be the bastion against such practices. The elegant jewelry stores of major cities proudly display platinum cocaine spoons for an up-to-date hostess to wear on a chain about her neck. This entertainment for the rich has received little comment from the arbiters of correct behavior who in the past spoke openly of the deplorable use of peyote among the Indian populace and the prevalance of cocaine use in the black community when it was a more available commodity. This volume makes no attempt to explain such transient patterns of drug use and the response that it evokes from critics.

In the past decade several excellent books on one or more aspects of psychoactive plants and their products have appeared. In addition to these we have a few fine volumes on psychopharmacology and anthropology as they relate to hallucinogenic plants. Few books have attempted an overview of narcotic plants as used in a broad generic sense. A spate of small handbooks has emerged from the alternative presses of the drug subculture, and a number of these are excellent for reason of presenting dosage levels of street drugs, others are deplorable in errant line drawings of plants and a jumble of misinformation. Unfortunately, one cannot be "almost correct" in identifying a plant that is intended for use in inducing an altered state of consciousness. Frequently, plants that are noxious poisons have been alleged to be mind altering.

In this book an attempt has been made to cover the narcotic plants of the world that have been used in a historical or contemporaneous context, to present the mode of use, the type of intoxication produced, a botanical explication, a chemical analysis of the psychoactive principle, and the geographical distribution of the plants. A thorough survey would require a presentation of encyclopaedic dimensions, but this volume encapsulates those plants that have had some part in shaping the history of peoples in diverse parts of the world. I have attempted to separate myth and legend from the known attributes of the plants surveyed. The neurophysiology and the neuropsychology of narcotic plants are well documented in volumes that probe the mechanisms of these altered states of consciousness, and no attempt is made to give such an explanation here. Likewise, the difficulty of separating learned behavior and psychodrama from behavior that is the result of the action of a narcotic on the nervous system is in the province of the anthropologist and the psychologist and has no place here. I might then say that this is an ethnobotanical survey of plants altering man's conscious state.

An explanation of the use of "narcotic" is in order, as this has medical definitions, legal definitions, and historical considerations that have shaped the interpretation and use of this word. If we adhere to a literal translation of the Greek word *ñarkotikos*, we may only include those plants producing a state of lethargy, torpor, or sleep. It becomes immediately evident that a number of plants termed narcotic have very different effects, often creating a state of nervous excitement or producing visions in the absence of any somnolence. I will use the term narcotic as it has been used by the United States Public Health Service to include those plants that are psychoactive regardless of the manifestation of this activity. We must keep in mind that terms such as "high" and "psychedelic" that have been broadly used are of recent vintage. When in 1957 Humphry Osmond first coined the word "psychedelic" he was using it to describe what he considered to be the "mind-expanding drugs." Not being totally convinced of such a thesis, I prefer to adopt the simpler term narcotic, which has a common meaning to large numbers of people, and not become embroiled in the controversy over enlightenment versus hedonism. In presenting the cultural context in which the plant is used I will describe the purpose ascribed to that plant by the people using it.

The most difficult task of this exposition is adopting a presentation that is sensible in organization and structure. Since no systematization of natural phenomena is natural, I will accept the inherently artificial nature of classification and utilize an order approximating that delineated by the famous toxicologist Lewis Lewin. The five categories of psychophysical states are: *excitantia, inebriantia, hypnotica, phantastica,* and *euphorica.* I will exclude the category of *euphorica* used by Lewin, for it included only two plants, *Papaver somniferum* and *Erythroxylum coca.* The former is perhaps best described as a hypnotic and the latter as a stimulant; thus they are best classified as *hypnotica* and *excitantia* respectively. I have added a chapter on tobacco, the enigmatic narcotic. These categories must overlap due to the complex chemistry of most of the plants in question. A number of the stimulants result in a deep somnolent state after the bout of extreme stimulation of the nervous system. Some of the hypnotics also provoke visions and thus become hallucinogens. Some of the known chemicals are actually neuroantagonists existing in the same plant.

"No civilization has found life tolerable without . . . the things that provide at least some brief escape from reality," writes Will Durant in his *Life of Ancient Greece.* And we have the observation from Dostoyevsky, that great chronicler of the complex passions of man, that "too much reason is a thorough-going madness." To such sage observations the botanist may append the observation that no flora of the world is without plants that can provide a respite from reality. Given the tortures of flesh and mind that are attendant on civilizations, it is understandable that man turns to chemicals that are capable of altering states of his consciousness, just as he turns from pain with a plant medicant. Whether these narcotics constitute a socially acceptable pastime or violate a legal or social sanction is a question that every civilization has had to answer, and the responses throughout history have been diverse. Consider the single plant *Cannabis,* described by the Emperor Shen-Nung as an important medicine in his pharmacopoeia that dates to an oral tradition going back to 2737 B.C. To the Hindus of India some centuries later it was "the heavenly guide." In the 1930's in the United States this same plant was called "the killer weed," "the destroyer of youth," and that which induced "reefer madness" culminating in murder and suicide. About four decades later in this country we find attitudes so changed that the plant is being investigated as a possible "recreational drug," and penalties for possession of small quantities are generally in the area of a misdemeanor. Quite obviously the psychological and physiological effects have not changed, but rather the judgements of society.

Apart from legal considerations and social approbation, many of the plants discussed in this book are of religious importance, have conditioned the architecture of certain cultures, have determined trade routes that later became the highways linking diverse areas, are medicants, have provided the basis for the new discipline of drug therapy, have been the foundation for masterpieces of music and writing, and a number have left the individual debilitated to the degree that he can no longer participate in his society at a meaningful level.

Despite all, man has used, and continues to use, narcotics to endure the duress of an otherwise intolerable existence. In the exudates and decoctions from trees and herbs, man has found principles that have permitted him to experience a kinship with the whole of creation. In exploring the flora of the world that has led to these altered states of consciousness, it is hoped that the reader will come closer to an appreciation of the total work of art that is man attempting to transcend the mundane.

ACKNOWLEDGMENTS

I wish to express my gratitude to Mrs. Frances Runyan for the exquisite paintings and drawings that she executed for this volume. Working with living material, herbarium specimens, and botanical descriptions, she has been able to re-create a host of narcotic plants, many of which have never been seen in publication. I also extend thanks to Miss Mary Butler and Mr. Joe Nakanishi for their paintings, which are extraordinary in both beauty and accuracy. My appreciation is extended to Mr. Robert Gustafson of the Botany Section of the Natural History Museum of Los Angeles. He has taken many of the photographs in this book (see photo credits), has located herbarium specimens and made loans possible, and has found many of the original descriptions of plants herein. My thanks are given to Mrs. Terri Kato Togiai, who typed this manuscript in its final form.

The following herbaria provided specimens without which this volume could not have been illustrated: The U.S. National Herbarium; The Herbarium of the University of California, Los Angeles; The Herbarium of the University of California, Berkeley; The Herbarium of the Natural History Museum of Los Angeles; The Herbarium of Rancho Santa Ana, Claremont, California; and The Herbarium, Kew Gardens, Richmond-Surrey.

Botanical gardens to be credited for their cooperation in making their facilities available for photographs are: The Los Angeles County Arboretum; The Gardens of the University of California, Los Angeles; The Huntington Gardens, Los Angeles; Kew Gardens, Richmond-Surrey; The Botanical Garden, Paris; The University Botanical Gardens, Vienna; The Botanical Gardens of Catania, Sicily; and the Tiger Balm Gardens, Hong Kong.

I wish to express my gratitude to Dr. Fred Truxal of the Life Sciences Division of the Natural History Museum of Los Angeles for making available drawings and photographs that are a part of the permanent collection of that institution. My appointment as a Research Associate at this institution has been most fulfilling.

Editorial direction by Mr. Robert Levine and Ms. Ilka Shore Cooper has been of great help. I thank both of them.

The Origins of
Narcotic Plant Use

Scientists generally agree that the use of narcotic plants dates to prehistory; however, the precise origins and patterns of use are disputed. In man's quest for food during the early nomadic period of his existence he would most certainly encounter some plants that were poisonous, others that would serve as adequate foods, and still others that produced bizarre and unusual effects by altering his consciousness. Among this latter group were those that would simultaneously sedate and relieve pain. In essence, man could be freed from his earthly bondage by these narcotic plants. To transcend the quest for food and to overcome pain and fear for a time would be as great a source of wonder as we can imagine early man encountering. How could he help but venerate such plants and regard them as mystical, and take them as substance for his set of religious beliefs? These would, in man's earliest civilizations, figure into his art as ornamentation on temples, as vessels or designs upon them, in his scepters and emblems of power, and especially in association with those figures regarded as deities.

This we find to be true in diverse cultures in which evidence for any early contact is lacking. Is this not a universal tendency among mankind? The sacred narcotic *Nymphaea caerulea* dear to Osiris is the crowning emblem of the Eighteenth Dynasty in ancient Egypt and predated that period by hundreds of years. In ancient Minoan cultures there are wondrous mace heads in the form of the opium poppy capsule, *Papaver somniferum*. The Incas had divinities that were fertility goddesses and the counterpart of Venus wearing the leaves of *Erythroxylum coca* as a headdress, so esteemed was this source of cocaine. The art of early civilizations in Guatemala and Vera Cruz presents us with stones that were formerly believed to be representative of phallic worship, but now we know them to be the sacred emblems of mushroom cults built upon several species of *Psilocybe*. Were not the earliest brewers in Mesopotamia and Egypt women of a priestly caste who produced the sacred libations of these civilizations? And what of the hymns of the ancient Vedic peoples of North India that sing the praises of the god-plant soma that transports and enlightens the worshiper who knows of this through the *Rig-Veda*.

Such a list would be too extensive to complete at this point, but it serves to indicate that whenever and wherever early man found a psychoactive plant he made it a part of his magical and religious set of beliefs, often venerating it and presenting it in symbolic form in many aspects of his art. Obviously, the plant had to be imbued with a divine spirit. It would then be reserved for magico-religious rites and would not become the object of hedonistic bouts of abandon. Wine as associated with drunkenness in a non-ritualistic context was not a part of early civilizations. In the *Symposium* of Xenophon we learn of the importance of wine in a ritual context, specifically the symposium and before it the recitation of the dithyrambos, the death and rebirth of the figure Dionysus. Even the chroniclers of drunken orgies associated with Dionysus are ignoring the ritual context of sparagmos and oomphagos. Likewise, the advent of Europeans in the New World brought them into conflict with those cultures that had found both the sacred mushroom *Psilocybe* and the narcotic cactus *Lophophora* being used under the name *teonanacatl*, or "flesh of the gods." This was too close to Christian tradition to be comfortably accommodated by missionaries. Such practices were condemned as pagan, perhaps because they were uncomfortably close to the religious practices of these conquistadors.

Personal ecstasis is perhaps one of the universal goals of man. That moment of revelation and enlightenment that sets him free may find its origins in plants. As civilizations grow there emerge those individuals who are able to experience and sometimes teach techniques of ecstasis. These are the shamans, the powerful ones. The shaman is able to teach "the way" as the result of his knowledge achieved through death and rebirth, this often occurring during a trance state. The first shamans were the first magi: they who enter the *magus*, a small enclosed space, to experience ecstasis. We have reason to believe that among the early Iranians this was achieved by way of smouldering hashish derived from *Cannabis*. The same material constituted the drug used to take away grief at the time of death among the Scythians, according to the Greek historian Herodotus. In shamanism the collective psyche of a people is brought into an ordered state. This revitalizes the culture, clarifies its world view, calms the collective psychoses, and relates the meaningful events of life in what may be termed a drug-induced psychodrama. That practice which in a contemporary society might be diagnosed as an illness was in earlier cults and tribes a solution to illness brought on by malevolent spirits. Thus we are compelled to see these practices in a historical and cultural context in order to understand them. What reason have we to believe that man has at some point ceased to seek personal revelation or ecstasis? As the religion of a society becomes more a part of the social order and loses its mystical content, we may expect more attuned individuals to seek that personal event that reveals to him his place in the world.

Several prominent writers discussing shamanism have failed to include the role of psychoactive plants in this phenomenon. If shamanism originated in the areas of Siberia and north Europe as indicated by many anthropologists, we may look to the mushroom *Amanita muscaria* as the agent that allows a man to "speak with spirits." In some accounts this may have happened some seven thousand years ago, devolving into the more sophisticated cults of Indo-Europeans some four thousand years ago. It would be this mushroom that called the first shaman to his profession of rendering the spirits of the world subservient to him. It is more difficult to believe that the repetitive states of melanotherapy and versotherapy alone induced this mystical vocation, or that they were the result of sensory deprivation, although all of these may result in trance states. The chemistry of the plant will determine the content of the psychic states realized in such a trance. If one is to have the imaginative power to reorder or restructure reality, it is not as likely to emerge from simple repetitive verse or movement as it is from ingesting a psychoactive substance. Botanists have made the observation that there are very few areas of the world that do not provide such plants as a part of the indigenous flora, and there are few of these that have not been used to achieve altered states of consciousness.

Notable among those writers on shamanism is Weston LaBarre, for he is in a distinguished minority in recognizing the important role that plants have played in the ecstatic experience. He is able to trace such practices to the Upper Paleolithic and Mesolithic hunting-gathering cultures of northeastern Asia at a date of some fifteen to twenty thousand years ago. La Barre asserts that some spiritually ungifted individuals, referring to autonomous ecstasis, are capable of visionary trances with pharmacodynamic help. He sees these as an important vehicle to shamanic ecstasy in prehistoric antiquity.

We need not restrict our attention to that category "phantastica" or the hallucinogens in documenting the ecstatic experience. In the cult of Dionysus it was the mentor of Dionysus, Silenus, who became prophetic when garlanded by mortals. Silenus relied upon inebriants to achieve this state. While neither Dionysus nor Silenus was anything more than a collective fiction among the ancient Greeks, their importance in an emblematic sense cannot be underestimated. The category of hypnotics or psychodysleptics is very amenable to that prophetic state that characterizes the shaman. The trance produced by *Mandragora*, the mandrake, certainly shaped the destinies of men for centuries in the Middle East and in western Europe. The plant itself was said to be prophetic. Effigies of the root carved into the form of a man were venerated throughout the Middle East, for it was believed that this root had the power to promote fertility. In Europe it was said that the spirit of the mandrake could materialize in various guises to do one's bidding. Excitantia would not seem to be a category lending itself to shamanic importance, but if we consider that cocoa is obtained from the plant that Linnaeus christened *Theobroma*, or literally "food of the gods," we have reason to recall that during the reign of Montezuma use of the cocoa bean was restricted to this man-god and his disciples. It was not in general circulation among the populace. *Theobroma* was believed to be an aphrodisiac with enormous generative powers. Likewise, with the euphoriant *Erythroxylum coca* we encounter a plant important above all others in the Incan ceremonies at the temple of the sun in Cuzco. The penitential suppliants could only approach the altar if they had coca in their mouths. Consider the suppliants at Delphi who could only approach the Delphic Oracle with leaves of *Laurus noblis* in their mouths.

These are but a few of those plants in diverse categories that have shaped man's thinking, formed a part of his religious beliefs, and conditioned the behavior of diverse societies. Collectively, the groups established by Lewin that constitute the various kinds of intoxications produced by narcotic plants may have had more importance in shaping civilizations than the other activities of mankind. It is in the temporary escape from totally rational thought and behavior that many of man's great achievements have been conceived. Revelation is not always the product of reason, and while Francisco Goya reminded us that the sleep of reason produces monsters, Dostoyevsky pointed out that too much reason becomes a kind of insanity. If the shaman is best characterized by "equilibrium," it is perhaps this delicate balance between the life of patterned rational thought and the ability to escape or transcend it that distinguishes the total man. Interludes of what some have called "expanded consciousness," whether induced by a plant drug or achieved by techniques of ecstasis, may be highly creative.

It has been characteristic of contemporary societies to legislate against the use of some psychoactive plants and their derivatives in the belief that such legislation will necessarily solve problems. It seems more reasonable to present factual information on these plants and chemicals derived from them in a historical context so that rational decisions may be made by an individual considering involvement in phytochemical experimentation. The knowledge that some of these may result in death, others in permanent neural damage, and others in nothing more than a transient harmless euphoria, will perhaps accomplish more than any form of prohibition. We have accepted the drug alcohol as a legal euphoriant despite its reputation for neural destruction resulting in total debilitation. The growing of tobacco, one of the most toxic plant drugs in current use, is subsidized by the federal government of the United States despite its link with cancer and other diseases. *Cannabis* laws are eroding in response to the knowledge that this plant is not the death-dealing weed that was the product of uninformed and misinformed legislators, rather a mild euphoriant. The object of this book is to clarify the history, chemistry, and current status of narcotic plants so that informed decisions may be made by legislators, teachers, and users of narcotic plants.

A Note of Caution
to the Reader

This book is an overview of the historical and contemporaneous use of narcotic plants throughout the world. It is not intended as a guide to the use of narcotics, but rather to serve the reader in an attempt to learn something of the botany of narcotic plants and to provide some perspective in an area clouded with misconceptions and misinformation.

A further note to readers: References in the text to figures (Fig.) are to black and white drawings, printed in the text; references to plates (Pl.) are to color illustrations appearing between pages 46 and 47.

HYPNOTICA, THE SEDATIVES AND TRANQUILIZERS

"Not poppy, nor mandragora,
Nor all the drowsy syrups of the world,
Shall ever medicine thee to that sweet sleep
Which thou ow'dst yesterday."

William Shakespeare
Othello, The Moor of Venice
Act III, Scene 3

IN ESTABLISHING THE CATEGORY of "hypnotica" among five classes of drugs, the German physiologist and toxicologist Lewis Lewin intended to include only those drugs that induced sleep. We are now aware that this category may be extended to characterize those chemicals that are capable of inducing a trance-like state and others that are tranquilizing without provoking sleep, a trance, or any stupor. All of these may be characterized as hypnotics or, more properly termed, psychodysleptics. The category is vast, as these plant drugs have been widely employed as medicants for many centuries. Under the name "soporific" they were common medicants in Europe and America long before the age of the tranquilizer. We may trace hypnotics in Western civilization to the early treatise of Theophrastus of Lesbos whose work *De Somnia*, or "Concerning Sleep," was the first treatise on sleep and ways of inducing it. His principal herb was the root of the mandrake, *Mandragora officinarum.* Sleeplessness has been one of the greatest diseases of man. This disease has found its remedies in those who practice the art of hypnosis as well as such non-drug remedies as that employed by King Xerxes, who had the chronicle of his empire read to him to induce sleep. I am particularly fond of the suggestion made by Lewin, "sometimes . . . medical books written by regular professors of the faculty are especially liable to produce sleep." The lack of sleep may be due to severe mental or physical anguish and is devastating in its effects. Shakespeare's King Henry IV cries for the gentle sleep that will steep his senses in forgetfulness, and he cannot understand why the "dull god" sleep lies with the vile man and leaves the couch of a king. Dis-ease is found in that most wretched of states, sleeplessness.

There is perhaps no better way to medicate disease than to remove the accompanying stress. In the opinion of many physicians it is the state of stress that permits diseases to ravage the weakened body. Behavioral psychologists and psychobiologists have shown the effect that crowding has on animals and people: stress and tension are gradually replaced by anxiety and aggression. Perhaps this explains why our "great civilizations" are being tranquilized into a more placid state by a variety of psychodysleptics. Lewin expressed concern in 1931 that those who had tasted the charms of sleep mediated by a hypnotic would be unable to resist habituation: "There is no hypnotic whose use is harmless, and medical men should take heart in order to prevent the increase of the already widespread evil of soporific consumption." Undoubtedly Lewin would view with horror the contemporaneous scene. The bromides of that era have been gradually replaced by the tranquilizers of meprobamate marketed under the trademark names of Miltown® and Equanil®, and more recently the compound diazepam sold under the registered name of Valium®. Useful in the treatment of alcoholism, in central nervous system abuse, for psychoses, in instances of hallucinations, it is an important therapeutic drug. Valium® is relatively safe, and overdosing and acute toxicity are rare when the drug is used alone. Unfortunately, used in combination with alcohol it may become lethal. Control is difficult, and the ten milligram tablets have found their way into the streets where they are sold for an average of one dollar apiece. This great anti-anxiety drug has found popularity in those individuals being wooed away from opiates by methadone. Methadone does not possess anti-anxiety properties as does heroin, so Valium® is used to remove these symptoms of stress.

Physicians who are not involved in psychotherapy have little recourse but to prescribe such a drug for anxiety-ridden patients. While we may deplore the extensive use of any such hypnotic, we must contemplate the alternative behavior of any society in the absence of these drugs and plants that have the property of removing stress, grief, anxiety, and the psychic wounds inflicted by civilization. Consumption of these tranquilizing and/or sedating pills in the United States alone is several billion each year. Is the motivation primarily hedonistic, or may we not find ourselves agreeing with the great philosopher Pascal, who is reported to have said that the greatest ailment of man is his inability to sit quietly in his chamber? Man in his ingenious search for that quietude has found in the stems, roots, leaves, and flowers of plants a solution to his historical dis-ease. Man does not always seek euphoria: he may, in Freudian terms, wish only to substitute the common misery of mankind for a state of neurotic despair. Can any attempt to escape into the realm of sleep or to allay anxiety really be considered deplorable? The historical antecedents for similar routes of escape take us back many millennia and require that we investigate diverse cultures in many areas of the world.

The ancient Greeks sought a condition of balance that freed them from the unpredictable disharmony of emotions. This state which they termed *ataraxia* was said to be obtainable through virtue and was the greatest good a man might realize. Is this not the same state sought in the great religions of the world? Variously called inner peace, the harmony of the spheres, inward calm, peace with one's self, and the divine harmony, it is the focal point of Buddhism, Taoism, Vedantist thought, and Christianity. It is a balance devoutly to be wished and not easily attained by "virtue." Although a distinction may be made between "genuine peace" and the delusion of the senses by a hypnotic, the effect upon the suffering individual is essentially the same. Thus, physicians now use the name ataraxis to characterize those drugs that merely tranquilize without producing drowsiness or sedation.

Establishing a quiescent state of mind is a form of therapy that harks back to the temple healers of ancient Greece who practiced their medicine in a temple-like sanitarium near fresh springs and who by a drug-induced hypnosis (accompanied by versotherapy and melanotherapy) worked their famous cures. Undoubtedly henbane (*Hyoscyamus* sp.), belladonna (*Atropa belladonna*), mandrake (*Mandragora offici-narum*), and opium poppies (*Papaver somniferum*) figured as their predominant medicants in various combinations. Asklepios, the divine healer, was named after the ancient Greek word for the rodent mole. The underground sanctuary at Epidauros had the interior design of a molehill and was the center for a cult of healers. The mysteries of the great god Dionysus were likewise recited in such labyrinthine underground chambers. These mysteries inculcated divination, a way of knowing that does not derive from intellectual prowess. Thus, healing in antiquity is revealed in certain states of consciousness. These may be induced by formulas repeated over many times, by ritual movements that are repeated endlessly, and by the consumption of a plant drug that will make the intellect subservient to the spirit and allow this divination and subsequent healing to take place.

A man who is sick has no *ataraxia*, that is to say, no psychic equilibrium, and it is the function of the healer to remove the spiritual imbalance so that the physical healing might take place. The first step in such a process would be to attain for the patient a kind of tranquility of mind that permits healing to occur. If we assume physicians of today to be correct in their assessment that about eighty per cent of all illness that they diagnose is psychosomatic, the procedures of the ancient Greek temple healers sound eminently logical and practical. Clean water, vegetable foods in modest amounts, and above all sedation induced by chanting ritual dithyrambs, and herbal sedatives were the substance of healing for these ancient practitioners.

In a not so altruistic manner, the ancient Aztecs found that there were hypnotics that could be given to a sacrificial victim that would not stupefy, but would sedate without any loss of motor coordination. This would permit a sacrificial victim to climb to the high altar for sacrifice in a trance-like state free of anxiety. It must be stated that the Aztecs had a number of hypnotics that were used as medicants. They served the same function as in ancient Greece, that is to say, they did not heal so much as they permitted healing to take place by removing stress and anxiety. The fortunate preservation of the Badianus Manuscript (Codex Barberini, Latin 241, in the Vatican Library) and its subsequent publication (1940) allows us to investigate the contents of an Aztec herbal dating to 1552. Plant medicants combined with incantations and charms constituted the primary office of healing. Ritual dance was also a part. Two types of healers were recognized, the *tepati* (from *teo-pàtli* indicating "divine medicine") and the *ticitl*, who was usually a sorcerer. Although animal parts and stones played a role in healing, a far more important role was played by plants, and Aztec herb gardens were extensive.

According to the account of a contemporary of Montezuma, doctor and historian Cervantes de Salazar, the old Montezuma had wondrous gardens filled with medicinal and aromatic herbs. "He ordered his physicians to make experiments with the medicinal herbs and to employ those best known and tried as remedies in healing the ills of the lords of his court." Chapter two of the Badianus Codex deals with, among other ailments, sleeplessness. Although all of the plants are illustrated, it is not often possible to interpret every one of them. Four identifications are made by the writer and illustrator, but of these only *tolouaxihuitl* is able to be positively identified as a kind of *Datura*, (Pl. 1). Such a plant would not only induce a profound sleep, but visionary experiences as well. We would probably characterize it as a hallucinogen. The chronicler Bernal Diaz wrote of the tobacco of Montezuma, which was mixed with unidentified herbs, and the gum of liquidambar or styrax (*Nicotiana* sp. and *Liquidambar straciflua*), which caused him to fall immediately into a deep sleep. For a cough the *tlacoxiloxochitl* was chewed or the root peeled and ground in water with honey. The botanical identification of this plant is *Calliandra anomala* (formerly known as *C. grandiflora*), and its feathery leaves and striking red flower with plumes of red filaments constitute a handsome shrub (Fig. 1). It may now be seen in Vera Cruz, Oaxaca, and south of Mexico City growing as a shrub or small tree. The Aztecs used it not only for coughs, eye diseases, dysentery, for a swollen anus and alimentary complaints, but they found incisions in the wood bark would yield a resin that collected in a dried form could be powdered with wood ash and inserted into the nostrils to induce a hypnotic sleep.

Teuvetli is a tree known to the Aztecs but remaining something of a mystery to contemporary botanists. We know that a tree by this name was incised to release its resins so that they might be used in ritual sacrifice. Slaves and captives had to climb to very high altars on these occasions and force was not appropriate to sacrificial ritual. It was necessary to induce a trance state that would not impair motor coordination and cause them to fall. We know little of this narcosis except that given this control of muscle combined with passive behavior it was most likely a hypnotic. *Bursera bipinnata (Elaphrium bipinnatum)* seems the most likely candidate for the mysterious tree (Fig. 2). *Bursera* species were used in diverse medical practices among the Aztecs. All of these have resin canals running through the bark and when slashed, a gummy resin is exuded. Leaves frequently spray a mist of volatile oils when broken. These gums and oils were applied directly to induced wounds before the ceremony so that a direct connection with the circulatory system of the blood might be established. This practice parallels that among the African bushmen who express the juice of a bulb of *Pancratium* (species unknown, but locally called *Kwashi*) into a wound on the forehead in order to provoke visual

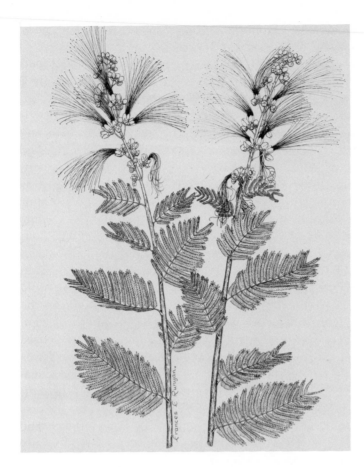

FIG. 1:
Calliandra anomala

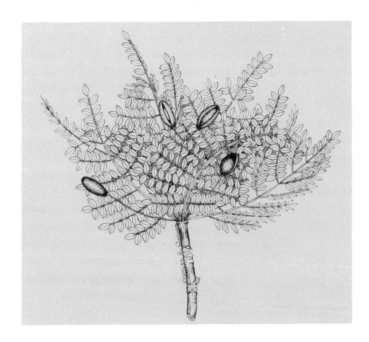

FIG. 2:
Bursera bipannata

5

hallucinations. In contemporary Mexico some species of *Bursera* (especially *B. penicillata*) are used to allay pain in instances of toothache.

The Badianus Codex provides us with an amazing array of Aztec medicinal herbs that were not only effective, but have not been replaced by other therapeutic agents even today. Some of these were not effective for the diseases that they were supposed to cure, but did have secondary effects of considerable interest. *Passiflora jorullensis* is a passionflower of considerable beauty and interest. It was known to the Aztecs as *coanenepilli* and was used to produce sweating, as a diuretic, against poisons and the bites of serpents (Pl. 2). It was also claimed to be a pain reliever. This red-flowered passionflower is clearly figured in the text of this ancient treatise in both foliage and flower. Very recent analysis of the foliage has shown it to contain harmol, harman, harmine, harmalol, harmaline, and passicol. The chemical harmine is also found in species of *Banisteriopsis* and *Peganum* and was once known as telepathine for reason of its peculiar ability to affect a contemplative state in which the eyes are closed and a slight feeling of euphoria is felt. Pain perception is diminished and a lowered sensitivity to outside stimuli is known. This is the drug obtained from the seed of *Peganum harmala* and used as a truth serum by the Germans during the Second World War. In this plant we have chemicals that are most allied to the true hallucinogens. Curiously, a recent group smoking the leaves of several species of *Passiflora* has found it a legal and effective substitute for *Cannabis* providing a similar euphoria.

This same early Aztec herbal makes note of an interesting use for the exotic tropical fruit *Casimiroa edulis* (Pl. 3). It is the seed rather than the fragrant fruit pulp that is used. The seeds are burned and powdered and used to induce sleep. Very recent assays of the powdered seed indicate the presence of N-Benzoyltyramine, methylhistamine, casimiroin, fagarine, and casimiroidine. The combination of these serves as an effective relaxant, and the plant known to the Aztecs as *cochiztzapotl* remains in use in Mexico today in areas where tranquilizers from drug companies are unknown. Fagarine slows down and regularizes heartbeats and is still used in medical practice to quiet uncontrolled muscle spasms and fibrillations.

Both the Chinese and the Japanese have used the Asiatic woody shrub *Actinidia polygama* under the names *ch'ang-chu* and *metatabi* respectively (Fig. 3). One primary use has been in zoos for the purpose of tranquilizing large cats. The volatile oils of the leaves of this plant contain metatabilacetone and actinidine, which might account for the effects. Chinese herb medicine prescribes *ch'ang-chu* in rice wine to further depress the limbic system and produce a sedative action. It would seem from experimentation that the drug acts upon the hippocampus and hypothalamus, producing some instances of visual distortion or hallucinations if large doses are consumed. As this leafy material is now often replacing catnip in imported toys for pet cats, these are more often opened and the contents smoked or made into a tea. The sprawling shrub also contains many of the oils found in catnip, which has been widely rumored to be a mild euphoriant. As yet no chemical substantiation exists for the plant *Nepeta cataria* as a hypnotic. "Chinese cat powder" has not caused any legislation to be formulated against it, as it is still not in widespread use and would appear to be nothing more than a mild hypnotic.

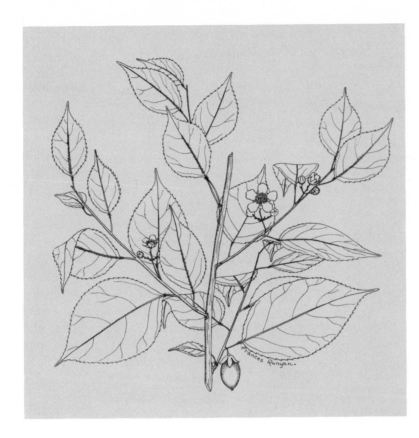

Fig.3:
Actinidia polygama

The origin of tranquilizers in the United States probably can be most accurately dated to the discovery in 1947 of an unidentified powder isolated from *Rauvolfia serpentina* (Pl. 4). This isolate had the ability to tranquilize laboratory animals without inducing any ataxia or stupor. In 1952 Dr. Schlitter and his colleagues isolated the crystalline substance responsible for this peculiar quiescence and named it reserpine. It not only tranquilizes, but also lowers blood pressure. Unlike many other hypnotics it takes several weeks for the total effects of reserpine to be realized, suggesting that it is in some way transformed in the body into secondary substances that produce the characteristic syndrome. It has been responsible for curing acute schizophrenia and migraine headaches and has assisted in withdrawal from opiates. It is believed that the origin of this breakthrough is only a few decades old, but to the contrary, it has an origin in India where it has been sold since antiquity under the name *sarpaganda*.

It has been written of the great leader Mahatma Gandhi that whenever he needed a period of introspection and detachment from the social milieu about him he drank tea of *sarpaganda* as holy men before him had done millennia earlier. The usual mode of use was to chew the root bark of this small shrub. Since it is the plant of contemplative introspection, it was appropriate to the holy men and would seem to indicate that it did them no harm, but rather freed them for the subliminal

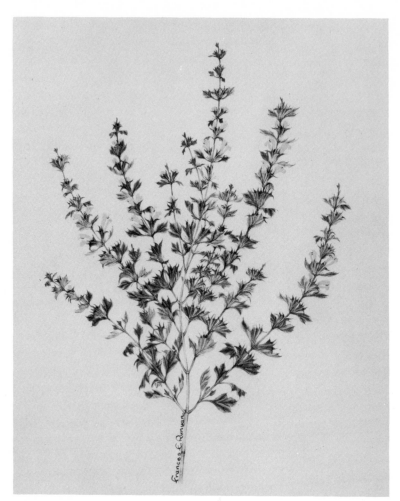

FIG. 4:
Lagochilus inebrians

thoughts that are so often more creative than channeled intellect. Since there are over fifty different alkaloids in the root of *Rauvolfia*, we may have reason to believe that the root bark is more effective than the single isolate reserpine. Over twenty-three species of *Rauvolfia* produce reserpine in addition to *Catharanthus roseus* and *Vinca major*. Reserpine acts on the sympathetic nervous system, depleting it of the neurotransmitter, norepinephrine; the sedating or hypnotic quality comes from some yet unidentified hypotensive activity.

India also provides us with one of the most widespread tranquilizers on that continent, but a plant that is virtually unknown to the rest of the world. *Withania somnifera* (Pl. 5) belongs to the nightshade family that provides the world with a plethora of medicines and drugs. This demure velvety green perennial plant seldom exceeds a few feet in height and would be altogether inconspicuous were it not for the bright red berries that develop within a translucent, enveloping calyx. *Withania*

8

has a considerable history in Africa as well. Liberians and Nigerians used the herb in its entirety by pulverizing the plant in oils and applying it externally to boils, swellings, and other painful parts. Internally it was used to tone the uterus after a miscarriage and in post-parturition difficulties. In Africa the leaves, and sometimes the entire plant, are sold under the name *ashwagandha,* and in addition to the aforesaid virtues, the material is claimed to rid the body of lice. Five subspecies of the herb are recognized in India and are found throughout the entire country. The dried root is sold in Indian markets as *kuthmithi,* as a tranquilizer for adults and unruly children or for those who suffer insomnia. The fruits, being high in saponins, find their way into a local soap. Although more than a dozen alkaloids have been isolated from the plant, the principal one is somniferine, which sedates with no undesirable side effects. The entire root bark in decoction is still more efficacious, however, than any single isolate. It would appear that there is a kind of synergistic effect when the several alkaloids combine in the body.

Russia has provided us with a hypnotic mint that grows on the steppes of Turkestan and is collected each October by the Uzbeks, Turkmen, Tartars, and Tajiks. *Lagochilus inebrians* is gathered in October by collecting the whitened, rather spiny branches that are then devoid of the small white flowers (Fig. 4). Silvery, opalescent stems bearing spiny bracts and calyxes are tied into bundles to hang upside down in homes throughout the long harsh winter. Curiously, the strength of the plant material increases upon drying, and a pleasant fragrance fills the room. For centuries the people in Central Asia have boiled the leaves and stems with sugar and honey to allay the bitter taste and from this produced a tea with strong powers of sedation. In addition to being useful as a sedative, it has antispasmodic and hypotensive qualities. Pharmacologists of the Soviet Union seem to have concentrated on hemostatic principles, as it is known to serve as an antihemorrhagic by reducing the permeability of blood vessels and aiding in the coagulation of blood. Allergies and skin disorders have been treated by this unusual shrub as well. The diterpene lagochiline has been assigned the function of achieving the sedation, but tests to ascertain this are lacking. *Tinctura lagochili* is in the official *Materia Medica* of Russia as well as the *Russian State Pharmacopoeia* (eighth edition). In 1945 Russian scientists isolated a polyhydric acid, lagochilin, from the leaves. It has been demonstrated that acetate derivatives of lagochilin are effective sedatives in humans in doses of as little as 0.03 grams. Much remains to be understood about the psychotropic activity of *Lagochilus,* and little has been done to investigate thirty-four other species native to central Asia, Persia, and Afghanistan.

Of all the sedating-tranquilizing-psychotropic plants known, the mandrake (*Mandragora officinarum*) has the most extensive and bizarre history (Pl. 6). This member of the nightshade family has been used as a painkiller, sedative, aphrodisiac, trance mediator, and poison. In heavy doses, extracts of this plant can create a stupor that resembles death. According to the "doctrine of signatures," every plant reveals in its parts the use for which it was intended; thus *Dentaria,* or toothwort, was good for toothache because of the tooth-like aspect of the underground rhizome. Herbalists writing on such matters capitalized on this peculiar notion, and it became a lucrative profession to harvest and sell plants of unusual form or herbs with some part that suggested a human member. Elaborate stories were concocted to keep the common man from harvesting certain medicinal plants, as this would destroy the inflated market.

The mandrake, having a root about a foot in length and sometimes branched so as to suggest the body of a man, would, of course, be the herb without equal. In keeping with the "doctrine of signatures" such a plant would medicate all of the ills of mankind. If the root did not conform to the shape of a man or a woman, it would be carved by charlatans to take on such an aspect. When the market was low, these same quacks would seek a surrogate, such as *Bryonia dioica*, and sell it to the unsuspecting victim. It was not uncommon to drill small holes over the surface of such a root and implant millet seeds. The root was then buried until the grains sprouted, after which time the whole thing was dried and had the aspect of a hairy little man. Both male and female forms were carved, and some of the females were shown to have children in their arms. A number of dessicated specimens unearthed at Antioch, Damascus, Constantinople, and environs had every conceivable form that an entrepreneur in an herb market might concoct. For the childless woman it was said that these roots used as talismans or amulets could overcome barrenness. We have in Genesis 30:14–16 the retelling of an ancient Babylonian myth in the story of Rachel and Leah. Rachel sought mandrakes from Leah's son to overcome the barrenness of her marriage with Jacob. It was not unusual for the women of the area of Palestine to bind a piece of mandrake root to their arm with a strip of leather to promote fecundity. We do not know the mode of use employed by Rachel, that is to say, whether it was talismanic or whether a medicant was made of the root. Both practices were common.

Mandrakes may have a yellow flower or a violet flower from which some botanists have sought to identify separate species (*M. autumnalis* and *M. vernalis*), but others believe the plant to have a single species with two flower colors and overlapping seasons of bloom. Both contain atropine, hyoscyamine, scopolamine and cuscohygrine (mandragorine). Other botanists have recognized as many as six species of *Mandragora*, all containing the above chemicals in varying proportions, making them the most powerful hypnotic plants of the Mediterranean region.

Theophrastus, the father of botany, wrote in his early treatises on sleep and in his compendium of plants: "One must make three circles around the mandragora with a sword while looking to the west. Another person must dance about the plant in circles reciting as much as he knows of love." Such a tale was to be elaborated upon with each passing century until the lore of the mandrake was burgeoning with contradictory statements. A synopsis of the legend as put forth by most writers of the sixteenth century would suggest the plant grew under the gallows where a man of virtue had been wrongly hanged and on the spot where his semen had fallen. Since the mandrake issues from the ground with great shrieks and groans, anyone hearing these would fall dead. The strategy suggested was to stop the ears with wool and beeswax; tie the neck of the plant to the neck of a dog with a stout rope; face the wind (west); throw meat to the dog, which, lurching, will pull the mandrake from the ground. In *War of the Jews*, Josephus added to this tale by advising the collector that the menstrual blood of a woman, or her urine, would aid in removing the root. He adds that it must then be hung from the arm or the collector will surely perish. Most of this he borrowed from Apuleius. The owner of a mandrake root was supposed to be able to call upon the spirit resident in this structure and make it do his bidding. Emperor Rudolph II of Germany surrounded himself with magicians, alchemists, and quacks of every sort. He owned two mandrake roots, which it is said he tended to as though they were his children.

Shakespeare found several occasions in which he was able to make effective dramatic use of mandrake legends. In *Romeo and Juliet* (Act IV, Scene III) Juliet reflects with trepidation on the spirits she might encounter upon awakening in her ancestors' tomb and their "shrieks like mandrakes 'torn out of the earth.' " Juliet believed that upon hearing these she might go mad. *King Henry VI* (Part II, Act III, Scene II) has the Duke of Suffolk utter a dread wish, "Would curses kill, as doth the mandrake's groan." In *Macbeth* (Act I, Scene III) Banquo asks, "have we eaten on the insane root that takes the reason prisoner?" These are but a few quotes from the venerable bard on the subject of the mandrake, but they serve to reveal its supposed attributes in seventeenth-century England: the mandrake supposedly caused insanity when pulled from the earth. Shakespeare's experience with botany and simpling was such that there is no reason to believe that he was deluded by such tales.

An early Arabic formulary tells of the mandrake used as a poison. An elaborate procedure was followed in decomposing the root: fermentation is induced until the root stinks (*sic*) and then another sixty days is allowed beyond this until the mass of pulp turns green and white. The pulp concealed in food or drink will cause loss of appetite, faintness, loss of breath, yellowing of the eyes, and itching of the entire body, trembling and shivering, fear of light, stomach pains, and finally epileptic seizures and death. If such a description conjures up great loathing and horror, avoid pursuing the cure, for it includes butter, honey, oatmeal, leaves and seed of rue, radish, dill, borax (at that time believed to be a stone from the head of a toad), mint leaves, anise, fennel seed, celery, absinthe, salt, natron, cinnamon, clove bark, nutmeg, wild ginger, mastic, etc. In brief, the victim of mandrake poisoning was given almost the entire list of spices, unguents, purgents, and herbs known at the time. It was this poison that was said to be used by the Duchess of Ferrara, Lucrezia Borgia, although history seems to have vindicated the poor girl.

In the tomb of Rameses III in Egypt as well as in several tombs of the Eighteenth Dynasty, we see the fruit of mandrake used emblematically with the opium poppy and the blue water lily in sacrificial wreaths, on the brows of mourners, and in offerings of food and vessels of liquid. It is one of the most frequent motifs on the "unguent vessels" that filled these tombs. In homes of this time small oil lamps burned before the dessicated roots of mandrakes. We have no doubt, then, that these were held in esteem by the ancient Egyptians. The legend of King Rā conquering Hawthor says that he put her into a deep sleep by mixing the beer of Helipolis with the blood of his people and with mandrake root. Its stupefying properties were well known.

Mandrake fruits were generally regarded as having the power to render a man speechless. It is not surprising that we encounter them under such names as Satan's apple, apples of the fool, apples of the genie, and Satan's testicles. The paired nature of the fruits undoubtedly accounts for the last attribute as well as the observation that the Arabs traded in these fruits with "mischief makers."

Mandrake leaves were read as tea leaves, used in infusions, applied to ulcers, scars, inflammations, and were even used as suppositories. As for the root bark, it was mixed with wine, lettuce seed, and mulberry leaves to form a potent anesthetic. It is recorded that the first volatile anesthetic was a sponge boiled in such a mixture and held under the face of the patient so that he might become anesthetized.

A very curious use for mandrake root was to make a bitter anesthetic known as *morion*. When crucifixions were common in the area of Palestine, the women there would offer a soporific sponge of this "gall" as palliative to the victims who were still alive on the crosses. In the 1880's a physician working with dogs and mandrake extracts suggested that the crucifixion of Christ did not bring about a demise, but with the aid of a sponge of *morion* he was put into a deep trance for three days. This was published in "The Asclepiad" and caused much controversy. Only recently a contemporary author has used this same thesis as the subject for a historical novel.

One of the most recent and intriguing exegeses on a hypnotic was suggested by Dr. Dobkin de Rios when writing on ritual uses of plants among the Maya. Having repeatedly encountered the water lily motif on Mayan ceremonial pottery in combination with the toad *Bufo marinus*, whose skin is hallucinogenic, she wondered at the possible properties of the water lily. In this regard I suggested that it had considerable antiquity in the northern parts of Africa as a hypnotic and was still used in some areas as a psychodysleptic. Her subsequent publication was followed by an independent analysis of *Nymphaea ampla* by Dr. Jose Diaz in which he found apomorphine-like compounds in the flowers as well as the already known nupharine and nupharidine. He further presented a mural at Bompak near Vera Cruz showing a shamanic ceremony involving the water lily and spoke of a contemporaneous use. Following these same pursuits, I was delving into the *Nymphaea caerulea* of the ancient Egyptians, since it is found in so many motifs in tomb painting, on unguent vessels, in stelae, and in association with almost every sacred artifact and occasion (Pl. 7). I was able to trace the first Old World use back to the Antilles as early as 1822, at which time *Nymphaea* was regarded as an effective substitute for opium. Many later reports confirmed that use. The aforementioned repeated association between this plant, the opium poppy (*Papaver somniferum*), and the mandrake in Egyptian tomb painting suggests that of the thousands of plants that might have been selected for depiction, only those of some ceremonial importance would have been chosen. All three are potent narcotics and would undoubtedly be used in any such rituals as something more than emblematic. We know that the unguent jars bear opium residues, indicating that they were not for water or perfume as previously suggested by Egyptologists. Further, *Nymphaea* flowers appear on most of these. The assertion that it is nothing more than a decorative motif is not reasonable in light of the total possible choices. The identification of the water lily with the figures of Rā, Atum, and Osiris, and the creation myths of the four cosmographies are evident. It is clear that the root was used as a famine food and the seed was milled into a crude flour. It is the flower proper that has historically been used as a narcotic. If this seems bizarre or untenable, consider that opium poppies producing narcotic latex in their seed capsules provide the non-narcotic poppy seed of commerce.

A recent report on the effects of apomorphine indicates that in low doses it is useful in overcoming schizophrenia, but in higher doses it is able to provoke psychotic episodes. Thus, the collective chemistry of *Nymphaea* species is such that it is easy to conceive of their importance in the shamanic structures of both Mayan and Egyptian civilizations.

Throughout the Pacific Islands, which figure so prominently in our romantic literature, there is cultivated a shrub that produces a slightly bitter, slightly soapy, aromatic resinous brew capable of inducing tranquility and ultimate somnolence. *Piper methysticum* is the binomial by which the botanist characterizes this plant, which is related to the black pepper of commerce (Fig. 5). In more traditional cultures, children are responsible for chewing the roots and lower stems of this

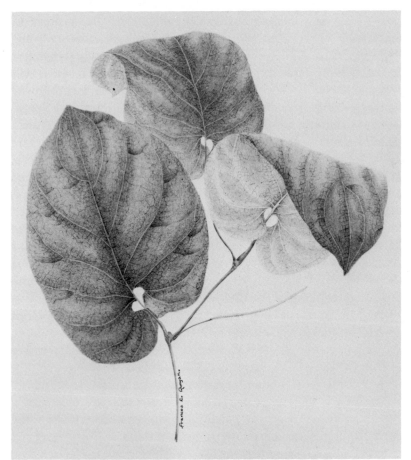

FIG. 5:
Piper methysticum

plant to produce the brew *kava (kavakava, keu, ava)*. The mouths of children are generally more disease free than those of adults, and their teeth are stronger. As they gnaw away a mouthful of the root, it is spit into a large wooden bowl. The alkaline saliva of the mouth with its salivary enzymes promotes the extraction of the active ingredients marindin and dihydromethylsticin. According to the native peoples of these islands, the brew produced in this manner is much tastier than that which is mechanically grated. Hygienic considerations have led the French and English to prohibit such chewing and spitting. Normally the saliva-root bark mixture is diluted by the addition of water, and the mixture is strained into coconut bowls. One half of such a bowl is enough to induce a state of well-being and a slight torpor which may terminate in a somnolence of several hours. Such a contentment seems to bring no cessation of reason, and active discussions occupy the participants. States of anxiety and restlessness have been recorded as reactions to large amounts of the astringent beverage. Such observations suggest that the exudate includes a more complex pattern of alkaloids, which might include some analeptics. It is now possible to purchase bags of dried and powdered root bark. A brew from this source lacks the aromatic properties of the freshly made *kava* and is not true to the flavor.

Oceanic cultures vary in the importance they attach to the use of *kava*. Samoa has perhaps the greatest historical use of the brew, and in Manua legend states that *kava* was first given by the Sun God to Tagaloa Ui, the first high chief of the Samoans. The legend begins with the sacrifice to the sun of a young virgin, Fituita, at the place where the sun rises. Her fate was to be that of other virgins who were each year devoured by the sun. However, one year a girl by the name of Ui was offered, and so great was her beauty that the sun took her to be his bride. When she became pregnant by this solar deity and wished to return for a visit with her people to give birth, consent was granted and she was sent flying through the sky at a tremendous speed. Unfortunately, she miscarried and the foetus fell into the ocean. All was not lost, for a hermit crab attended to it, along with a plover and a shrike. The boy grew under the guidance of this unlikely trio into Tagaloa Ui. It was he who taught mortals how to make *kava*, as well as the reverential ceremony that surrounds its use. Pava, the first mortal to participate in the ceremony, had a son who laughed at the antics of his father as he attempted to prepare this brew for Tagaloa Ui. In god-like wrath Tagaloa Ui cut the son into two pieces to the dismay of Pava, and then proceeded to instruct Pava in the correct manner of preparing *kava*. After a wooden bowl was filled with *kava*, Pava offered it to Tagaloa Ui, who did not drink it, but poured it on half of Pava's dead son and uttered *"soifua,"* or life. At this pronouncement the boy was made whole again and Pava clapped his hands in joy. With the admonition that *kava* pertains to high chiefs and is sacred, Tagaloa Ui took his leave. Rituals since that day involve the pronouncement and clapping of hands.

This elaborate myth contains all of man's relationship to sun, sky, water, earth, plants, and animals as well as attributes of the "Divine Being," the mortal self, birth, death, resurrection, marriage, mystical spirit flight, and shamanic transformation. It seems to embody the essence of many myths in diverse areas of the world that also include a psychoactive plant. It parallels the Osirian mysteries with no transcultural contact. This ritual use of *kava* remains most intact today in Samoa, but in the Oceanic area in general *kava*-bars are not uncommon and are becoming the coffeehouses of this great area.

Even though members of the genus *Datura* are properly discussed as mediators of hallucinations, they have also been used historically as powerful sedatives. When Cristoval Acosta visited India in 1578, he learned that seeds of *Datura* were used by "mundane ladies" (prostitutes) to sedate their clients so that they might be easily robbed. Many of them had been taken into prostitution at an early age by similar sedation and kidnapping. In ancient Greece the priests of Apollo used *Datura* to achieve subliminal, sedated, prophetic states. It would appear from seed remains in the Temple of the Sun in Sagomozo that *D. sanguinea* served the same purpose in magico-divinatory rites in which the prophet was in a semi-somnolent state. Thus, it is not easy to assign *Datura* to only one category of narcosis. Temple priests of the Incas used *D. fatuosa* in performing surgery as a way of sedating their patients so that they would feel no pain and would not thrash about. This would appear to be one of the first instances in the New World in which a priest administered a medicine rather than taking it himself. Similar uses were found in ancient China and *Datura* was known under the name *man-t'o-lo.*

In the Darien and Choco territory of Central America, an extract of *Datura* seed was used to stupefy children so that they would wander about in a semi-somnolent state until they fell into a coma. It was believed that where they fell gold would be found. The scopolamine and hyoscyamine in most species of *Datura* may be used to explain the effects.

Europe for centuries used hypotensive drugs in instances of what was variously described as hysteria, nervous affliction, mania, etc. Some of these demonstrably relieve man's inquietude and others seem to have an undeserved historical use. One of the best known of these is the dried roots and rhizomes of the hellebore, *Veratrum album*, which only recently has been shown to contain the steroids proveratrine A and B which act on the afferent side of the sympathetic nervous system (Fig. 6). Equally effective, and historically praised, is the wild valerian (*Valeriana officinalis*) of the British Isles and throughout much of Europe (Fig. 7). The rootstock has a disagreeable odor, but when boiled (one ounce to one pint of water) it makes a strong nervine that was famous for promoting sleep. The herbalist Gerard claims that this was the root of which Dioscorides wrote as effective against poisons and pestilence. Gerard knew the plant as "setwall," which he stated "is in such veneration amongst them [the poor people] that no broths, pottage or physicall means are worth anything if setwall were not at an end." Apparently the root had an immense popularity that superseded the physical desire for food. The plant continues to be used as one of Europe's principal sedatives as well as the active principle, monoterpene valepotriotes.

The passionflower of the Aztecs mentioned earlier has a parallel in *Passiflora incarnata*, which has not figured into ritual, but was used for many years as a nervine and now has found its way into sleeping pills. Religious persons found the entire passion of Christ displayed in the floral configuration of this attractive plant. Although this added nothing to its efficacy, it certainly enhanced its popularity.

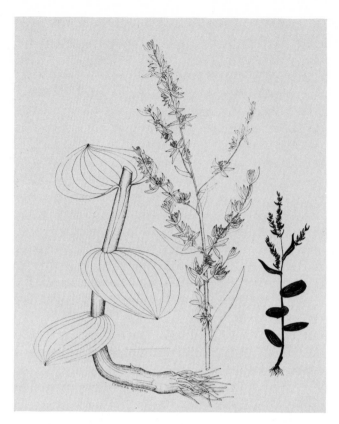

Fɪɢ. 6:
Veratrum album

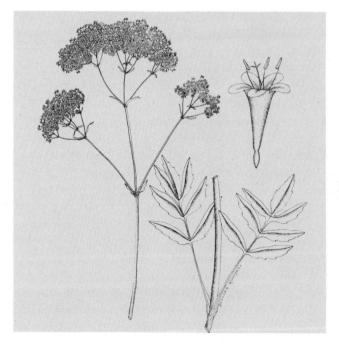

Fɪɢ. 7:
Valeriana officinalis

Orchids are rarely thought of as anything more than ornamental, but in both Europe and America the sedating effects of the root of the lady's slipper orchid were well known. The name derives from "Our Lady's slipper," referring to the shoe of the Virgin Mary. The saccate labellum and its resemblance to female genitalia is inescapable; thus we have *Cypridedium calceolarus* prescribed most often for hysteria, weakness of women, and female disorders (Pl. 8). As a nervine it was prepared by chopping the roots into powder and adding this to two parts, by weight, of alcohol. Placed in a dark area for eight days in a stoppered bottle, a crimson fluid is obtained, which was described by one of the leading nineteenth-century herbalists as having "a nauseous fecal odor." What price sleep! This harkens to a most unusual practice among the Ayurvedic shamans. It had long been observed that bees gathering nectar from *Vanda roxburghii*, one of the loveliest of orchids, would soon fall into a stupor on the ground below (Fig. 8). Ayurvedic shamans used the flower in a decoction to achieve the hypnotic narcosis of their office, permitting them a transcendent state of being.

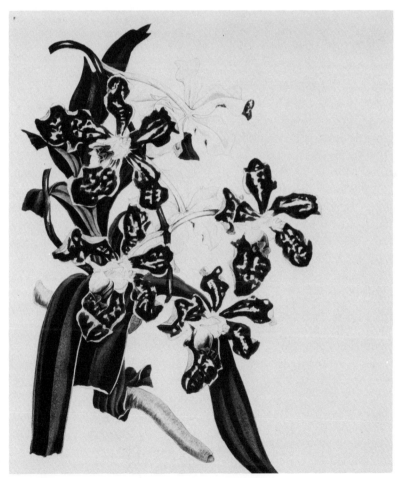

FIG. 8: *Vanda roxburghii*

17

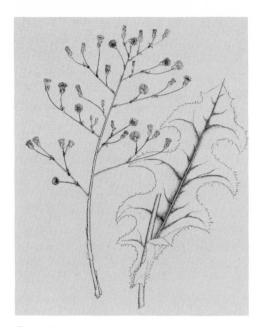

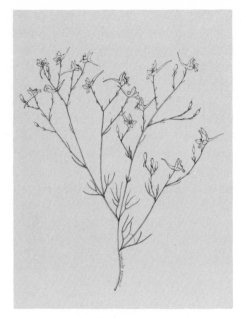

FIG. 9: *Lactuca virosa*

FIG. 10: *Delphinium consolida (Consolida regalis)*

A plant as common as lettuce is not likely to be suspect in any category of psychotropic plants, but it was known for a long time that the bitter leaves of the wild lettuces, *Lactuca virosa* and *L. quercina*, possessed a latex that could be reduced to a dark, gummy mass that would exhibit opium-like properties (Fig. 9). Lettuce-opium was the name given to the dried latex, and the active principle was said to be lactucarium. More recently, popular magazines representing the drug subculture have had full-page advertisements for lettuce-opium in various forms, as the plant is a "legal high" according to the advertisers. A "legal low" would be more to the point, since lactucarium has a sedating effect and is not a euphoriant.

In England *Delphinium consolida* had long been known as King's consound (from the Latin *consolida*, "to console in time of distress") (Fig. 10). It has a fine sedating quality and constituted a basic home remedy. Similarly, in northern California the Capella Indians prized the magnificent red delphinium that encrusts a naked stem in late spring. The root of this larkspur that is naturalized from England was pulled in the late spring and used to induce sleep in children and ailing adults as well as stupefying one's foes and impairing their judgement.

Apart from the use of *Avena* grains to sedate, a practice that is questionable, there are few members of the grass family that are psychoactive. The darnel of the Bible is not a grass but is the fungus *Claviceps purpurea* that establishes itself on the plant, replacing the grain. There are, however, two grasses in the United States that do intoxicate. One of these is to be found growing around the upper Rio Grande in the Sacramento–White Mountain region. Known by the name *popoton sacaton*, this grass suggests an Aztec origin; the hahuatl-derived name means "sleepy grass."

Popoton sacaton is botanically *Stipa vaseyi* and is most common in Guatemala, where it is also used for inducing sleep (Fig. 11). A related species in the same genus, *Stipa viridula*, grows as a perennial herb on the eastern ranges of the coast mountains in California: it too has a narcotic effect on the spinal cord and brain, but I am unable to find any historical context for its use.

In northwestern United States, *Lycopodium selago*, known as wolf's foot and club moss, is common in the temperate forests where it thrives in moisture, shade, and rich humus (Fig. 12). Three stems of this plant, which are only a few inches tall, induce a mild hypnotic narcosis, while eight of these will result in a total stupor or even a comatose state. The Potawatomis gathered *L. obscurum* var. *dendroideum* while the Flambeau Ojibwas utilized *L. compalanatum*. It is worthy to note that *Lycopodium selago* was known to the Druids and used by them as well as by most ancient physicians in Europe. The knowledge that this is an active narcotic poison should be enough to dissuade those who would look to this as a recreational drug. Purgation and catharsis are part of the physiological response to this plant that was the *Muscus terrestris* of earlier physicians.

Among the lower Chinook and the Quinault of the Pacific Northwest Indians, *Arctostaphylos uva-ursi* was used in two ways (Pl. 9). Berries of this shrub are effective in allaying appetite, but the leaves were of greater importance, for they constituted the smoking substance called *kinnikinnick* (or *kinikinik*). This practice spread into Canada and became a major item of exchange with other Indian groups and with the settlers who mixed it with their limited supplies of tobacco from *Nicotiana tabacum* to form *sagack-homi*, known among some western hunters as

Fig. 11: *Stipa vaseyi (S. robusta)*   Fig. 12: *Lycopodium selago*

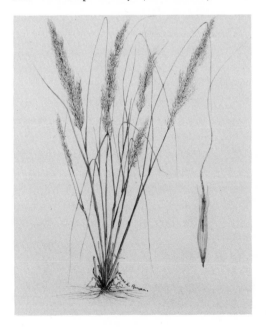

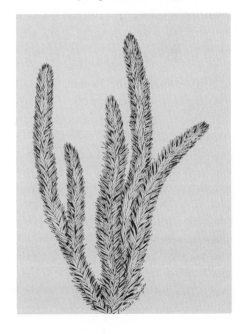

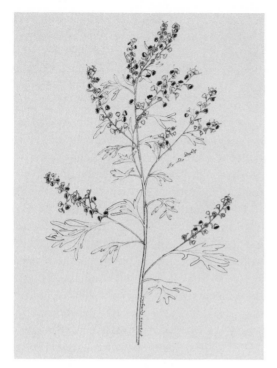

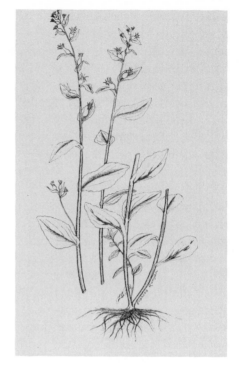

Fig. 13: *Artemisia absinthium*   Fig. 14: *Lobelia inflata*

larb. While this was the principal smoking mixture of several groups of Indians, there is no indication that any of them employed it with the regularity with which tobacco is used. Among the Menomini and Thompson indians, the bear-berry leaves were made into an astringent to strengthen the bladder and kidneys, but these same leaves were also smoked. There are records of individuals becoming so intoxicated by this experience that they would fall into a fire and remain immobile. Was it an experience of induced ecstasis, a hedonistic venture, or a medication? The question remains unanswered except for the evidence that the settlers were drawn to it as they were to their tobacco.

Unfortunately the common name uva-ursi has been used to denote such diverse genera as *Ledum, Rhododendron, Loiseleuria, Gaylussacia, Arctostaphylos,* and *Vaccinium;* some authors have even included *Arbutus unedo,* whose fruits are made into a narcotic wine. Early records show that the Shakers of Groton, Massachusetts, ignored the uva-ursi common to their area and would go forty or fifty miles to Danvers to gather leaves of *Vaccinium vitis-idoea.* Uva-ursi dates to the thirteenth century when the physicians of Myddfai used it as an astringent. Clusius described it in 1601 as the plant of Galen and indicated it as a hemostatic; it was admitted into the London Pharmacopoeia in 1763 and continues to be sold in leaf form even today.

At an unspecified early date the settlers brought *Artemisia absinthium* from Europe to the gardens of the colonies to provide a medicant for stomach ailments and bronchitis (Fig.13). The volatile oils in this herb are absinthin and absinthol, which have the capacity to produce a benumbing intoxication and to destroy neural synapses. Oils of *Artemisia absinthium* combined with anise, coriander, and hyssop formed the narcotic alcoholic beverage Absinth, which was so popular as a "tonic drink" at the end of the nineteenth century in Europe. Because it causes permanent neural damage, this beverage is now illegal.

Lobelia cardinalis was prized by the Cherokees as an anti-spasmodic, and *L. inflata* was known to the settlers as Indian tobacco (Fig. 14). It was presumably smoked for asthma, bronchitis, and similar respiratory disorders as well as being made into a tea-like infusion. The common red lobelia, *L. cardinalis*, used among the Cherokees, was noted by the famous American botanico-pharmacologist Millspaugh to have an acrid property and to function as a nervine. All of the species of *Lobelia* cause a giddiness in acting upon the central nervous system. One would be tempted to ascribe the action to the principal ingredient, lobeline, but this goes unsubstantiated. The roots of *L. cardinalis* and *L. siphilitica* (thought to be a cure for syphilis at one time) were used by the Meskwakis as love potions. Millspaugh noted the power of *L. inflata* to "relax the whole system," but disapproved of the practice established by a Dr. Samuel Thomson, who claimed it to be a curative in all disorders. It should be stated that in large doses it acts as a neural poison.

Too many plants were known as "Indian tobacco" to give the name any real validity. We do know that when tobacco was in short supply a number of surrogates were found. One interesting false-tobacco is *Gnaphalium polycephalum*, a common annual herb with floccose-woolly leaves and branches and floral heads with thin, overlapping bracts (Fig. 15). The entire plant has a pleasant fragrance and is quite viscid to the touch. The flowers were often stuffed into the pillows of consumptives, as they were believed to have a quieting effect. Some of the common names betray the use: "ladies tobacco" is perhaps the most popular name applied to several species of the genus. The leaves were often smoked by women as they were considered milder than tobacco and more fragrant. Early experiments by homeopaths indicated that the leaves and flowers produce "giddiness, especially on rising" and a "dull, heavy expression of countenance."

Phytolacca americana is known to every child in the East and Midwest who has mistakenly eaten pokeberries and experienced the extreme cramping and dysentery that the purple fruit provokes (Pl. 10). The root of this plant had long been used in China (*P. acinosa*) for reason of its similarity to the form of mandrake and ginseng (*Panax quinquefolium*) and the hypnotic qualities of its rather large root. Poke greens were a common potherb in the early spring in most households in the eastern United States, and in the fall the root of this tall herbaceous perennial was dug and found its way into many home remedies, despite the knowledge that an overdose leads to a paralysis of the respiratory system and ultimately death may ensue. Nonetheless, it continued in use as "cancer-root" and for many of the same problems for which belladonna was used. *Phytolacca americana (P. decandra)* was also used by the Indians of the Pacific Southwest for its narcotic properties. Romero, who has written extensively on plant use in this area, extols the virtues of the plant and states that it is to be preferred to morphine, opium, and cocaine. He further notes that it was very important in Indian formulas. It found its way into the British *Extra Pharmacopoeia* of 1804. Despite stupor, dullness, giddiness, and vertigo, Millspaugh spoke of *Phytolacca* as "one of the most important of the purely American plants."

The use of the buckeye *Aesculus* species dates to the writings of Matthiolus in his letters on medicine. The most common practice was to use the bark or ripe hulled fruits placed in alcohol and permitted to steep for eight days (Fig. 16). The astringent, orange tincture would then be given to treat fevers. The fruit of *Aesculus pavia* was used by aboriginal peoples in stupefying fish. The most interesting use was put forth by a Dr. McDowell, who used the powdered testa, or seed coat, of the fruit as an opium substitute. According to this authority, ten grains of this powder are equal in potency to three grains of opium. Certainly, any opium substitute is worth further inquiry. The fate of this remedy was to fall into obscurity, for it did not appear in the *U.S. Pharmacopoeia* nor in the *Eclectic Materia Medica*. The belief in *Aesculus* seed was so considerable that it was customary for persons to carry the nuts in their pockets, believing this would cure a host of diseases. It is worthy of note that *Aesculus chinensis* has had a long-standing popularity in China, where it is used against palsy and rheumatism. Of *Aesculus glabra*, a Professor E. M. Hale wrote in 1877 of its action on the nervous system to cause "confusion of mind, vertigo, stupefaction and coma." These are symptoms that are accompanied by gastrointestinal complaints.

FIG. 15: *Gnaphalium polycephalum*   FIG. 16: *Aesculus californica*

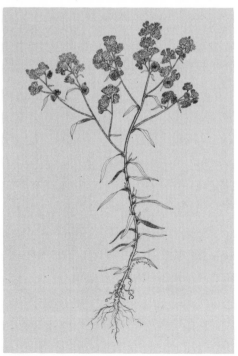

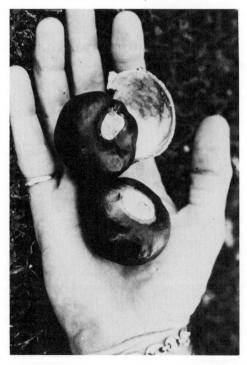

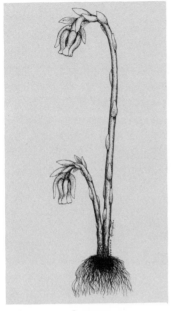

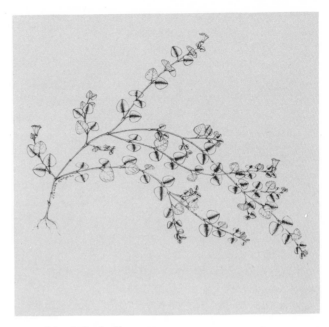

FIG. 17:
Monotropa uniflora

FIG. 18: *Mitchella repens*

In the nineteenth century Dr. John King recommended another plant native to woodlands of the temperate United States as an effective substitute for opium. *Monotropa uniflora* was long valued by Native Americans for its fresh juice, which was used on inflamed eyes and would overcome nervous irritability, including fits and spasms, without any disagreeable side effects being recorded (Fig. 17). This demure saprophytic herb used to be common in beech and maple hardwood forests but is considerably endangered at this time. Its mysterious appearance in the spring under these trees as a white ghost-like apparition has earned it the name "corpse-plant." It has a cold, waxy, clammy quality and upon being touched turns black. It enjoyed considerable popularity as an opium substitute without ever entering any materia medica.

The Menomini used the aforementioned *Cypripedium* orchids as a nervine, especially *C. acaule.* Their troubles with insomnia and similar disorders are attested to by another favorite soporific which they employed with some regularity, the partridge berry. A tea made of the berry of *Mitchella repens,* an attractive creeping plant of the madder family, has a very definite sedating action on the nervous system (Fig. 18). Sometimes the entire plant was consumed or made into a tincture that had the odor of Scotch whisky laced with wintergreen. Although it never became official in any dispensatory other than the *Eclectic Materia Medica* as *extractum mitchellae* and *syrupus mitchellae,* it is worthy of attention. The plant is still fairly common in forests of temperate United States and Canada.

These same forests support *Actaea alba,* or white cohosh, and *Cimicifuga racemosa,* or black cohosh (Figs. 19 and 20). Although disposed in different genera,

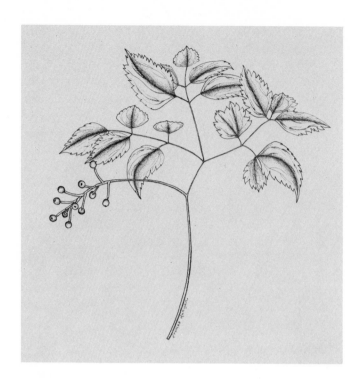

FIG. 19:
Actaea alba

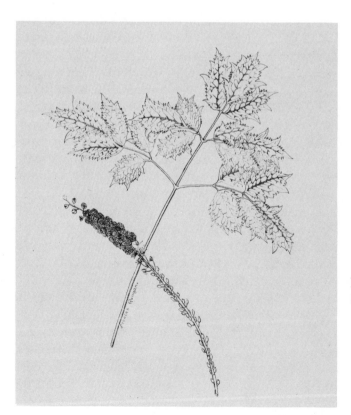

FIG. 20:
Cimicifuga racemosa

these two plants resemble one another in both morphology and physiological action. Once referred to by mid-nineteenth-century doctors as useful only to "Indians and quacks," it came into common use and entered the *U.S. Pharmacopoeia* because of its effective action on nerve centers. Millspaugh states that it became a favorite among "all tribes of the aborigines." In utilizing *Actaea alba*, a tincture is made of the whole plant, but only the pulverized root of *Cimicifuga racemosa* is employed as a nervine and for "relaxing hysteria." An insoluble resin has been characterized as cimicifugin or macrotin, but neither seems to properly characterize the active principle.

Solanum nigrum, the black nightshade, has a history dating to Dioscorides, the Greek botanist and physician of the first century who recognized the medicinal value of this cosmopolitan member of the nightshade family (Pl. 11). Arabs applied the bruised leaves to burns and similar skin diseases. Throughout the Middle Ages this plant never went out of popularity as a sedative, anti-spasmodic, for bronchitis and asthma, etc. In Dalmatia the root was fried in butter and eaten to produce sleep, while in Bohemia the flowering plant was hung over the cradle of infants to lull them to sleep. The latter was not a wise practice, as the unripe berries contain enough solanine to poison a child. As a hypnotic this plant has been said to equal the various species of lettuce that provide lactucarium. The usual mode of use was to make a tincture of the whole plant. This rancid-smelling fluid is disagreeable to the taste, being both bitter and acrid. The Rappahannocks used it for sleeplessness by steeping a few leaves or the entire plant in a large quantity of water. An overdose causes vertigo, vomiting, a cold sweat, and death may ensue. When the fruit has matured into a deep purple-black berry, the solanine is gone and the fruit is delicious. Having had a black nightshade pie, I can attest to its splendid flavor, which is not unlike that of huckleberries (*Vaccinium*).

Yellow Jasmine refers to *Gelsemium sempervirens* of the southeastern United States (Pl. 12). This yellow-flowered vine is not related to the true jasmine of Europe. There is dispute as to whether the virtues of the roots and flowers as a narcotic were first discovered by the natives of North Carolina or by one of the early physicians among the settlers. John Brickell mentions it as one of the plants useful in a host of diseases, and his writing did not originate with him but is mostly an account of Indian uses of native herbs. *Gelsemium* became official in all materia medica of the United States.

The greatest hypnotic in history is opium, which is derived from *Papaver somniferum* (Pl. 13). In the latex of its unripe capsules, the addictive alkaloids morphine, codeine, and thebaine are found. These are phenanthrene derivatives and are unlike the non-addictive alkaloids such as papaverine, which exert their principal action on smooth muscle tissue. Heroin is a synthetic derivative of morphine. There is a tendency to think of the widespread use of opiates as a contemporary phenomenon, whereas it may be traced to the most ancient civilizations. The popularity of opiates over the many other hypnotics mentioned is because of the unparalleled efficacy of these in allaying pain and providing a feeling of well-being. About eighty per cent of those individuals who use opiates seem to fall into a pattern of physiological addiction that is difficult to cure. When one suffers from extreme physical or psycho-social pain, taking recourse to a euphoriant without equal is understandable. The "junkie life style" is a characterization of a social pattern set up by criminalization of the addict that forces him into a life of crime. The behavior that is most intolerable in a society is created by that very society. The issues are not simple in the least, and the National Institute of Mental Health is supporting many programs investigating treatment modalities. Laudable though this is, relatively little federal support is given to the study of causal aspects of the problem. Cures are not effected by removal of the drug, but by destroying the circumstances leading to its use. There are too many sources of opiates throughout the world to hope for a destruction of the source of opium, and the techniques of smuggling are too diverse to expect to eliminate the influx of heroin.

A historical overview of opiates may provide some insights into contemporary usage. The presence of the opium poppy in the ancient Near East is a matter of some contention. Those who repeat the often printed figure that opium dates to 4000 B.C. in Sumeria should look deeper into history, for Sumeria did not exist at that date except as a sort of subunit of ancient Babylonia-Assyria. All of the opium poppies, and there are numerous forms with respect to features of the plant, seem to be derivatives of the wild poppy *Papaver segetaria*. Basically, all opium poppies are cultigens. The form of the capsule in *Papaver somniferum* is exceedingly diverse, as is its size. Flowers appear in numerous colors of white, lavender, pink, red, and with or without markings on the petals. This has created controversy in interpreting the motifs in Assyrian and Egyptian antiquity. It has been suggested by Krikorian, a noted authority on the poppy, that some of the forms identified in this ancient civilization as poppies are portrayals of pomegranates. A number of artifacts from ancient Assyria, however, would suggest the poppy capsule in identifiable form in this area in antiquity.

Poppies were known to the ancient Egyptians and figure prominently in their art in tomb paintings, mace heads, and in the earliest medical papyri. It was a plant of great power and was highly venerated. We have found traces of opiates in those glorious "unguent jars" of the Eighteenth to Twenty-eighth dynasties, leading us to believe that perhaps the "unguent" or "perfume" was in reality a narcotic potion. The frequency of the additional rendering of mandrake and the narcotic water lily on these vessels reinforces this contention. The form of the capsule is quite beautiful and naturally was emulated in vessels of all sorts (Fig. 21). The Persians knew the opium poppy and cultivated five or six varieties. In ancient Greece, *nepenthes*, "that potent destroyer of grief," would seem to be the opium poppy that had come to the Greeks by way of the Egyptians. In Greek and Minoan art the poppy motif is found on signet rings, on coins, in hairpins, in jewelry of all sorts. Theophrastus knew of it as a sleep-inducing drug in 300 B.C., and his observations were repeated by Pliny in the first century A.D. with added observations on opium poisoning. The Greeks consecrated the poppy to Nyx, goddess of night, Morpheus, son of Hypnos and god of dreams, and Thanatos, god of death (Fig. 22). They summarized all of its properties in the deities to whom it was offered. Opium spread throughout the Arab empire after the seventh century. It was undoubtedly used both as a medicant and for those overburdened with grief and care. We know that

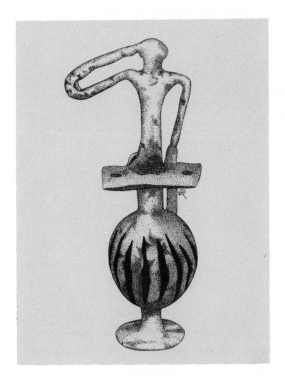

FIG. 21: Opium poppy motif,
Greek bronze

FIG. 22: Nyx distributing
poppy capsules

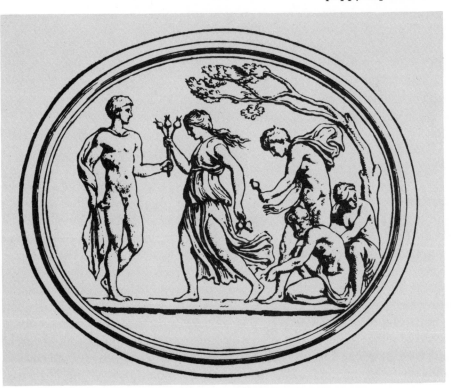

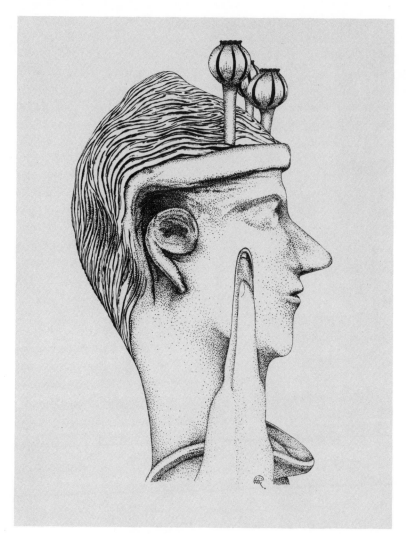

FIG. 23: Terra cotta head from Knossos bearing a corona of incised poppy capsules

the great physician Avicenna died of opium intoxication in Persia in the year 1037.

In the eighth century B.C. Hesiod wrote of a town near Corinth named Mekone, or "town of the poppy." That poppies could be so important is attested to by the famous terra cotta bust of a goddess at Knossos, Crete, bearing a corona of incised poppies (Fig. 23). While Hippocrates, the famed Greek physician (460–377 B.C.), advocated poppy wine as a medicine, Erasistrates and Diagoras of Melos warned against this medicant. The usual mode of consumption was to drink the hypnotic gummy latex dissolved in wine (Fig. 24). Many Greek women were seemingly addicted to the philtre that Helen offered to Telemachus, which would "lull pain and bring forgetfulness of sorrow." Almost every Greek writer finds some occasion to mention the opium poppy or *nepenthes*, and the same may be said of the early

Romans. The reputation that the poppy root was a potent aphrodisiac was spread by the Greeks, but originated among the Assyrians and Babylonians. This erroneous tale no doubt hastened the spread of the poppy.

Capsules from this great classical civilization are almost always figured with incisions, indicating that they have been deprived of their latex in order to obtain the opiates. It has been a tradition for women and children to practice the subtle art of cutting the capsules while they are still green and doing so without injuring the seed within, for that is an equally important food crop. Shortly after the fall of the petals there is a period of about ten days in which all of this must be accomplished. Most poppies reach maximum production of narcotic latex about three days after the corolla has fallen to the ground. A several-bladed knife on a ring provides an ideal instrument for the surgery. The latex collection is accomplished by simply peeling the dark gum from the capsule and working it into the ball that is to become the crude opium of commerce.

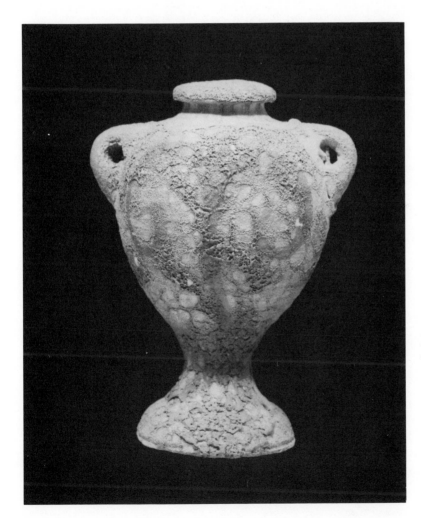

FIG. 24: Opium vessel —Knossos

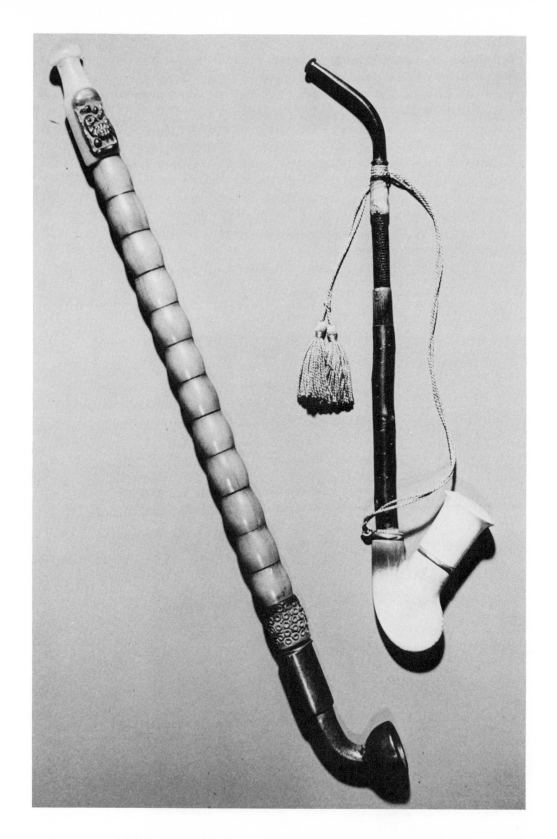

It is a false notion that China spread the cult of opium use, for in China *Papaver somniferum* was grown principally as an ornamental garden plant until the nineteenth century, with occasional use in medicine. It was Java and Formosa in the East and India in the West that carried the practice to China. In an attempt to prohibit the use of opiates, the Chinese government forbade the import of opium, leading to the First Opium War (1839–42), which brought China and Great Britain into conflict. The battle was a losing one, for addicts in China had risen to the millions: a trend that continued until 1906 when an imperial edict forbade the use of opium and the growing of the opium poppy. Opium was not manufactured in China before 1853, and the crude opium that the East India Company smuggled into Canton was so despised by the Chinese that they called it "Foreign Black Mud."

Although the usual mode of consumption of opiates at this time is by way of intravenous injections, opiates may be eaten, sniffed, drunk, or smoked. In Asia smoking *chandu*, a specially prepared opiate dried over a flame, is a common practice. A small lump of *chandu* is rolled between the fingers over a lamp and then deposited into the bowl of a pipe (Fig. 25). *Chandu* burns to yield an intoxicating smoke and leaves a highly toxic dross in the pipe bowl. This residue is in turn smoked by those who cannot afford the luxury of *chandu*, and their fate is to die of this within a very few years.

In Europe of the nineteenth century the use of opiates was so widespread that no stigma was attached to the regular use of this narcotic. Thomas de Quincey was addicted by the age of twenty as the result of using laudanum, which is a tincture of opiates with various additives. In his *Confessions of an English Opium-eater*, he spoke of opium ruining the natural power of life but at the same time providing "preternatural paroxysms of intermitting power." De Quincey wrote of the growing popularity of opium in the English working class, whose wages were not enough to provide them with ale or spirits, so that they had to indulge in the less expensive habit of buying two- and three-grain pills of opium. He appended to this, "I do not readily believe that any man, having once tasted the divine luxuries of opium, will afterward descend to the gross and mortal enjoyments of alcohol."

Elizabeth Barrett Browning had an opium addiction as did Coleridge, who is said to have written *Kubla Khan* under the influence of the drug. Berlioz romanticized the opium reverie in his *Symphonie Fantastique.* There is little doubt that the nineteenth-century view of opiates was quite different than it is today. Doctors created an immense addiction by prescribing opiates to women for diseases such as hemicrania, insomnia, hysteria and "the vapors." At the turn of the century in America, a survey in San Francisco revealed that opium addiction was not a problem of the impoverished, the Chinese, or the black, but it was the middle-class white American woman who ranked highest in this habit. At this time one American in four hundred was involved in some opium habit. Peculiarly, there was no outcry from legislators and no menace seemed apparent in this involvement with

FIG. 25: Opium pipes

the poppy. Some fears were being expressed as early as the mid-nineteenth century concerning morphine, which had been isolated from crude opium in 1803. Ironically, in 1898 heroin was placed on the market as "the perfect drug," for it was advertised as "more potent, less harmful and non-addicting." It was seven years later that one text dared to assert that these attributes of heroin were "perhaps not entirely correct."

It seems strange that with the tremendous amount of research on morphine and its substitutes there is still a great deal that goes unexplained with respect to the specific action. We do know that there is a general decrease in brain arousal to pain and that respiration is depressed. One other prominent effect is to decrease digestive juice flow and increase the amount of water removed from the intestinal tract. It is the suppression of tension, anxiety, and pain that best accounts for the use of opiates. The feelings of anxiety that some choose to include in the syndrome of effects seems to be related to the absence of opiates or the fear that they will not be forthcoming.

Assuming a daily injection of heroin in a dose of one-quarter to one-sixth grain, the average person will become addicted within a two-week period. Unfortunately, the initial euphoria is not repeatable unless the dose is increased each time until a tolerance level develops. From that period onward the motivation is purely to prevent the horrors of withdrawal—in which every orifice of the body flows, muscles twitch and contract, the colon writhes, and the bowel evacuates. Vomiting becomes so severe that blood vessels rupture and blood is spewed about. A general sensation of tremendous pain makes the situation unbearable.

The only viable alternative to opiates seems to be methadone, a synthetic addictive opiate that may be taken orally and is administered under governmental supervision. It does not produce euphoria, there is less depression of the respiratory system, and the side effects are much like those of heroin: constipation, sexual inadequacy or delayed ejaculations, an increase in the frequency of hallucinations, numbness in the arms and legs, and other less serious effects. There is one major benefit of such a program that substitutes one addictive substance for another addictive compound, and that is the social issue. Methadone patients may lead normal lives of a constructive nature rather than turning to crime to support a habit that may cost over three hundred dollars every day. The social good is evident; there is much debate over the issue of substituting new opiates for old.

As indicated earlier, several plant substitutes for opium have been known for a considerable period and yet none seems quite effective in that the properties found in most of these do little more than remove pain and depress the central nervous system. Lettuce opium (not an opiate at all) and the testa of the buckeye relieve pain and sedate without euphoria. In Assam, Burma, and Thailand the leaves of the bush *Mitragyna speciosa*, also known as *kratom*, are used and are best treated as hallucinogenic. Seeds of the Tula tree, also called *bekaro (Pterygota alata)* are used in Sylhet and Andamas in West India as a substitute for opiates, with considerable success according to the people of this area and in Pakistan. A report from north India suggests that Ayurvedic medical men have an enormous success in curing this habit by employing a tincture of oats *(Avena sativa)*. One of the most interesting and neglected reports was made at the turn of the century and emanated from San Francisco. The *American Pharmacist* for the year 1898 reported that boiling the entire mature plant of *Sonchus oleraceus*, the common sowthistle, produced a brew that was shown to be effective in getting the Chinese of that area away from opium. It is doubly curious because the young shoots of this plant are a common potherb eaten in England and the United States. It would seem that, given the current crisis levels of addiction to opiates, especially heroin, any and all of these deserve some very serious attention from pharmacologists and biochemists.

Bittergrass of Mexico is not a grass, but a composite *(Calea zacatechichi)* common around Tehuantepec, Oaxaca (Fig. 26). In 1968 a naturalist, Thomas MacDougall, working among the Chontal Indians, reported a "secret" plant that is made into a tea or infusion and consumed in solitude while a cigarette of the same leaves is smoked. This produces a feeling of well-being that continues for one or more days. It is said that *Calea* promotes repose and one hears one's own heart and

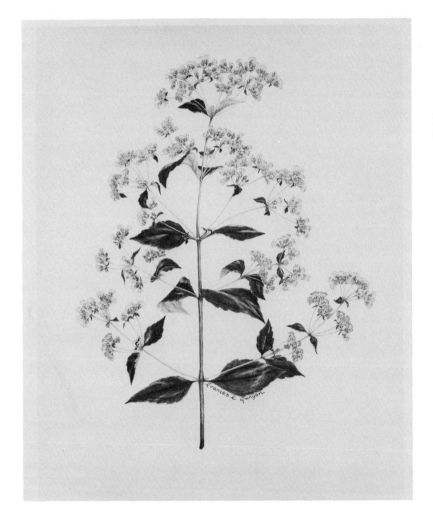

FIG. 26:
Calea zacatechichi

pulse beating. There is no indication of true hallucinogenic effects. The use by sabio-curanderos for clarification of the senses of *Calea* under the name *thle pela kano* does not imply a visionary experience, but the term means "leaf of god" to the Chontales.

Upon the suggestion of Dr. Michael Harner, James Fadiman investigated the use among the Yaqui shamans of North Mexico of a peculiar smoking "tobacco" of *Genista canariensis*, Scotch broom (Pl. 14). Information from a Yaqui shaman provided the mode by which the flowers were prepared. Having been sealed in a glass bottle for ten days, the small yellow flowers were removed and dried over low heat; they had not lost their color in this process and had not fermented or been subjected to the action of fungi. Rolled into cigarettes, these were smoked. Less than one cigarette produced a relaxed feeling with no subsequent depression. Several cigarettes produced longer lasting and more intense feelings of relaxation, intellectual clarity, and physical ease coupled with psychological arousal and alertness. Although no distortions or hallucinations were reported, a heightened awareness of color and contrast was noted. Just before sleeping, a period of extensive hypnogogic imagery was experienced by one of the participants. No deleterious side effects were realized when the flowers were of the correct plant and properly prepared. These flowers may be confused with those of *Spartium junceum*, which contains the toxin spartenine. *Genista* has trifoliate, persistent, villous leaves; *Spartium* has glabrous, linear leaves and has a more barren appearance.

TOBACCO, THE ENIGMATIC NARCOTIC

"For thy sake, Tobacco, I
Would do any thing but die."

Charles Lamb
A Farewell to Tobacco

"A custome lathsome to the eye, hateful to the nose,
harmefull to the braine, dangerous to the lungs, and
the blacke stinking fume thereof, neerest resembling
the horrible Stigian smoke of the pit that is bottomlesse."

King James I
A Counterblaste to Tobacco *(1604)*

ALTHOUGH IT IS DIFFICULT to position tobacco with respect to other psychoactive plants, the effects of large dosages suggest it to be a powerful narcotic capable of causing delusions and hallucinations. The dilemma of characterizing tobacco is that it may act as a stimulant, a depressant, a tranquilizer, or a hallucinogen. Lewin and several subsequent writers have treated tobacco as a stimulant, but nicotine, the pyridine alkaloid primarily responsible for tobacco's physiological action, has a complex action related to dosage levels. A typical cigarette provides enough nicotine to act on the central nervous system to cause cortical arousal. In the autonomic nervous system it mimics acetylcholine, stimulating neurotransmission. Nicotine, however, is not rapidly broken down, and less than two per cent of all smokers are occasional smokers, or more precisely are non-habituated. Thus, nicotine accumulates and acts as a neural block with respect to the transmission of new information. Sensory receptors are stimulated and then blocked. Acute nicotine poisoning causes tremors, convulsions, respiratory paralysis, coma, delusions, and death.

Nicotine, in the form of tobacco, is the most addictive drug in common use. As early as 1597 the famed herbalist John Gerard noted in his *Herbal* that "drinking tobacco," as smoking was then called, led to addiction: "Some use to drink it for wantonnesse or rather custome, and cannot forbeare it, no not in the midst of their dinner. . . ." Gerard observed the same frantic hourly inhalation that characterizes the contemporary addiction to tobacco. It is one of the few drugs that gives the user no respite, and it is far easier to develop a nicotine dependence than an alcohol or barbituate dependence. Some users from Synanon, a rehabilitation center, who have also been involved in a heroin habit, have found it is easier to kick heroin than tobacco. Major factors responsible for widespread addiction are as follows: social approbation, governmental subsidies for growers of this narcotic, enormous publicity campaigns with political lobby groups behind them, and the manipulation of advertising by way of sexually oriented advertisements. The 1979 report of the Surgeon General's Advisory Committee on Smoking and Health listed an impressive array of deleterious effects of and diseases caused by, or exacerbated by tobacco smoke, and this list is still growing: lung and other cancers, shortened life expectancy, heart disease, emphysema, bronchitis, more aborted and stillborn babies, underdeveloped babies, increased susceptibility to contagious disease, etc. Equally significant is the finding that those individuals who are forced to be in the environment of the smoker are compelled to suffer many of these same diseases. It is the only addiction that is forced upon non-addicted individuals with the sanction of the federal government that has so piously, and yet aggressively, worked to eliminate drugs of lesser addictive properties. A young attorney, John F. Banzhaf III, has given up his private legal practice to fight to reduce the rate of addiction among smokers, to protect non-smokers, and to upset the present balance of power in Washington legislation that gives support to the producers and promoters of this dangerous narcotic.

Tobacco juice and smoke was probably the first narcotic used in South America and was one of the most important components of the *materia medica* of the payés, or medicine men. Rochefort, in his history of the Antilles, describes the role of tobacco in the making of a medicine man. The eldest son of a payé inherits his father's office only after several weeks of initiation into the mysteries of curing, interpreting, and predicting (divining). Since tobacco plays such an important role in these rituals, the novice is dosed with tobacco until it no longer functions as an emetic. When practicing his art, or sullen craft, the payé evokes his own familiar demon by the dual attraction of chanting and smoking tobacco. Smoke blown upon a sick person is supposed to effect a magical cure. Payés, like the curanderos of Mexico, intoxicate themselves in order to divine and predict. The tobacco may be taken in the form of juice expressed from the plant and drunk in large amounts until a stupor ensues in which divination can be carried out and the source of the illness revealed and defeated. If smoke is to be blown upon the patient, a common payé practice is to hold the cigar, which is about two feet long, with the lighted end in the mouth; the smoke is blown out the opposite end. This practice survives today in several areas of South America. In 1526 Captain Gonzalo Fernandez de Oviedo y Valdés in his *General and Natural History of the Indies* wrote of a herb called "tobaco" used by the Indians of this island "in order to go out of their senses." He also noted, "the Indians considered this herb very precious and grew it in their gardens . . . taking this herb and its smoke was not only a healthy, but also a very holy thing to do."

Richard Spruce, who studied the lore of the Indians of the Amazon basin in the early 1850's, commented that while the payés of that region are often unskilled in their practices, this lack of skill is compensated for by the faith of their patients. Further, the practices of these medicine men are certainly no more ridiculous, and far less dangerous, than those described by Molière in his satires of French doctors. We would do well to remember that in the payé tradition the doctor consumes the medicine. In the history of Western medicine the extensive bloodletting, consumption of toxins, caustic enemas, mercury-lard steam baths, ingestion of precious stones, and so forth are hardly more laudable than the smoke cures of the Amazon basin.

Tobacco used by the Indians of the Amazon region was probably *Nicotiana tabacum*, but of a more potent variety than is now usually grown, as attested to by the stupor and delirium caused by smoking or drinking the juice of the herb (Pl. 15). This plant grows several feet high, arising from a basal rosette of glandular leaves and terminating in a cluster of pale pink, tubular flowers. The heavy musky scent of these viscid glandular hairs has been used not only in primitive medicines, but as a base for perfumes as well.

On the north coast of Cuba, only a few miles from Antilla, is the city of Gibara where Columbus landed on November 5, 1492. The esteemed admiral sent several of his men, laden with gifts, into the interior where he believed the king of these people was living. Hoping to be regaled by stories of gold and jewels, one can imagine his astonishment when the Spaniards returned, not with jewels, but with tales of men and women inserting into their nostrils smouldering rolls of leaves which they called *tobacos*. These *tobacos*, which we would call cigars, were inserted into one nostril, ignited with a firebrand, and inhaled two or three times. It is hard to imagine that within a few decades there were more Spaniards converted to smoking than Indians converted to Christianity. Similarly, when British navigators attempted to settle Virginia, they found the Indians smoking cigars, pipes, and chewing and snuffing. Walter Raleigh, one of these navigators, was so fascinated that he took pipes, tobacco, and an Indian to demonstrate these curious practices in London. The plant taken to England was a low-growing, glandular herb-bearing cluster of green to yellow-green flowers. We know this plant today as *Nicotiana rustica*, a very potent member of the genus (Pl. 16).

Tobacco conquered the English as surely as it had the Spaniards, and soon the London Company was sending African slaves to Virginia to clear forests, to plant and cultivate the weed. However, it was not *N. rustica* that was grown, but its Brazilian cousin, *N. tabacum*. As Virginia and Maryland were depleted of their forests, a tobacco aristocracy grew rapidly, and by 1640 the annual export to England alone was over one million pounds to satisfy the demands of almost 7,500 tobacco shops in London alone. At the time of the American Revolution, debts of colonial planters to British firms ran into several millions of dollars, a debt that was later to be settled for a fraction of the amount owed. Among the tobacco aristocracy were Thomas Jefferson and Patrick Henry.

The reaction among the English was not all favorable. A notable figure speaking out against "so vile and stinking a custome" was King James I. It was to him a "filthie noveltie, so basely grounded, so foolishly received. . . ." Papal edicts were issued against the use of this plant through the sixteenth and seventeenth centuries. As the herb spread to the Near East, various forms of torture were used to dissuade potential smokers. China went so far as to use beheading to turn away those who would import tobacco into China.

Nicotiana tabacum spread throughout the world with such rapidity in part because of its habituating properties, but also for reason of sailors' tales that affirmed it to be a potent aphrodisiac. Sailors told of the women of Nicaragua who smoked this weed and displayed an ardor undreamed of. It was probably this rumor that clinched the popularity of smoking among the women of Europe. Perhaps this is the reason why an ex-Franciscan monk, André Thevet, experienced such success in introducing tobacco to the French court in 1579. Thevet brought seed from what is now Rio de Janeiro to France in 1556. It was known to the Brazilians as *petun* and *petum*. In a volume of 1557 known by the first word of its nineteen-word title, *Singularitez . . .* , Thevet described various things from "Antarctic France, otherwise called America." Among his commentaries, we have those relating to *petun*: "this herb may not be taken without harm, for its smoke causes perspiration, and weakness and even makes the users fall into syncopes, and this I personally experienced. This is not as strange as it seems, for there are many other fruits [sic] offending the human brain, although, if eaten, they have a good and pleasant taste. . . ." This did not discourage Thevet from introducing the plant and publishing an account in which he takes credit for this act and casts aspersions on an unnamed individual who claimed to have introduced this plant at an earlier date, and who further had the audacity to give his name to the plant. The culprit was none other than Jean Nicot, French Ambassador to Portugal, who had brought from the king's prison in Portugal an herb of unusual properties. This plant could reputedly, if snuffed up the nose, relieve severe headaches. A gift of the powdered leaves and seed was sent by Nicot from his garden to Catherine de Medici in 1560. Catherine suffered severe headaches, probably migraines, and was pleased to receive the powder which was to be used as a snuff. It was not *Nicotiana tabacum* that was received by the Queen, but *N. rustica*. Ultimately it was the contribution of Thevet that was to conquer France and not the weed of Nicot. A battle of words over the primacy of introduction ensued and Nicot, having considerably greater status than Thevet, published with other scholars in 1573 a dictionary in which this entry is to be found:

> *Nicotaine: a herb of marvellous virtue against all wounds, ulcers, face*
> *ulcers and similar things, which M. Jean Nicot, Ambassador to the King*
> *of Portugal, sent to France and from whom it has derived its name.*

Nicholas Monardes, writing as Physician of Seville in 1557 in his book *Joyfull Newes Out of The Newe Founde Worlde*, wrote "Of the Tabaco, and of His Greate Vertues" speaking of the plant growing in Mexico (Newe Spaine), which was probably *N. rustica*. Monardes used the Aztec-derived name of *pecielt*, which he took from *picietl* (or *piciyetl*), and spoke of the wondrous effects wrought by the plant under the influence of the devil, whom he described as a deceiver and one who "hath the knowledge of the vertue of Hearbes."

> One of the merveilles of this Hearbe, and that whiche doeth bryng moste admiration, is the maner how the priests of the Indias did use it . . . he toke certain leaves of the Tabaco, and caste theim into the fire, and did receive the smoke of them at his mouthe, and at his nose with a cane, and in takyng of it, he fell doune uppon the grounde, as a dedde manne, and remainyng so, accordyng to the quantitie of the smoke that he had taken, and when the hearbe had doen his woorke, he did revive and awake, and gave theim their aunsweres, accordyng to the visions, and illusions which he sawe. . . .

This constitutes one of the earliest accounts of New World shamanism involving a narcotic as revealed by a European. He repeatedly insists that "the Devill" gives counsel to those who are in a tobacco trance. It indicates to us that the tobacco used was very likely the potent *N. rustica*.

Linnaeus, when compiling his binomial system, probably consulted the dictionary entry made by Nicot, for he dubbed all of the tobaccos and their relatives with the generic epithet, *Nicotiana*. Thevet seems to have suffered an injustice in this apellation, but the harm seems slight if one considers Spanish volumes that predate both of these individuals in speaking of tobacco. The contributions of the two were quite different: Thevet introduced *Nicotiana tabacum* with the idea of its becoming a popular plant to smoke, while Nicot introduced *N. rustica* in the belief that it was a medicinal snuff. The popularity of snuff throughout Europe shortly after its introduction cannot be attributed to medical properties, for it has no real use in medicine. It is the plant of Nicot that we now use for making a variety of insecticides.

In the Aztec idea of medicine, *Nicotiana rustica* figured prominently. Medicine being allied with purification and power as well as trance states for the purpose of divination, the herb *picietl* was ideal. Centuries before the Conquest, the Aztecs used *N. rustica* in cleansing rituals that still persist among some descendents of these people today. Leaves of *picietl* were dried and powdered and this bright green dust was rubbed over the temples, forearms, stomach, and legs. Such a ceremonial ablution was called *limpia*. In addition to this ritual cleansing, *picietl* was an important masticatory. A wad of leaves was chewed with a bit of lime in much the same way as coca leaves are used in Peru. A quid of *picietl* fortified by lime was soon relegated to the area between the teeth and cheek, where it could be sucked for some considerable time. The Aztecs also used *N. tabacum*, another *yetl* or tobacco, which they called *quauhyetl*. The latter came from Brazil and the manner of use from the people of the Andes. Zealous Christian friars and priests wrote extensively against the use of *yetl* by these people while concurrently the monastery gardens of Europe (especially France) abounded in tobacco, and many an abbé carried a snuffbox. It was again the association between the plant and religious belief and practice that confounded the clergy.

The Badianus Codex speaks of *picietl* being mixed with bark, leaves, several herbs, salt, pepper, crushed stone, ashes, and bitter water for rumbling of the abdomen or diarrhea. The manner in which this medicine was used was characteristic of several New World Indian tribes. The aqueous mixture was put into an animal's excised scrotum that had been attached to a horn with the tip removed. This provided an ideal clyster or enema. The horn or a hollowed plant stem was inserted into the anus and the scrotum of liquid was squeezed. In the instance of repeated afflictions, the *picietl* was made into a strong potion and the sick person was obliged to drink it. The process began with purging via the juice of *Agave*, which would cause vomiting. On the third or fourth day the patient was to drink juice of *Iresine calea* and the exudates of two other unidentified plants in hot water. This was followed by another plant that induced purging (appearing to be a *Mimulus* sp.) steeped in wine. The patient was given a bath and anointed with *Agave* juice and then experienced two more enemas. The first enema was of a *Begonia* species and the second, administered a few days later, was of *piciyetl (picietl)* mixed with black pepper, salt, and water. This was designed to produce inebriation. Sensitive translators have spoken of "anointing the abdomen," but in the original it is stated, "*Alvus bis clystere purgandus est. . . .*"

Tobacco is described by Rafael Karsten as the medicine of sorcerers and indispensable at the great tobacco feasts of the men and women among the head-hunting Jibaros of eastern Ecuador and Peru. The observations of Karsten were made in the early 1930's and present us with a fascinating account of a ceremony that is probably thousands of years old. Among these people tobacco is the most important and most indispensable medicine. It has been identified as *Nicotiana ondulata*. The Jibaros usually take tobacco in the form of a liquid made by boiling the plant or by chewing the leaves and expectorating into a large bowl. The latter process provides medicine for the great feasts and is particularly sacred. An old man of the tribe chews the leaf, and he also must administer the brew. Men receive tobacco juice through the nostrils and the women through the mouth. After two or three doses, the participants turn pale, tremble, become giddy, and fall into a drugged sleep with peculiar dreams. The reasons listed by Karsten are as a prophylactic against evil and disease, to increase the body's magical powers, and as a narcotic to produce dreams.

Johannes Wilbert reported on a contemporaneous tobacco ceremony involving shamanic ecstasis among the Warao Indians of Venezuela, in which tobacco smoke from enormous cigars is used to propitiate spirits and to induce trances among the priest-shamans. Tobacco smoke can be used to intercept the flight of spirits. An important statement made by Wilbert and too often overlooked by ethnobotanists concerns the effects of tobacco: "Even if it is not one of the 'true' hallucinogens from the botanist's or pharmacologist's point of view, tobacco is often conceptually and functionally indistinguishable from them." Wilbert sees tobacco as essential to the functioning of the Waraos' social and psychic equilibrium. He believes that he is able to find origins for this Warao shamanism in Mesolithic and even Paleolithic Asia, introduced into the Americas 15,000 to 20,000 years ago!

Charles B. Heiser, a specialist on Solanaceous plants, has pointed out that both

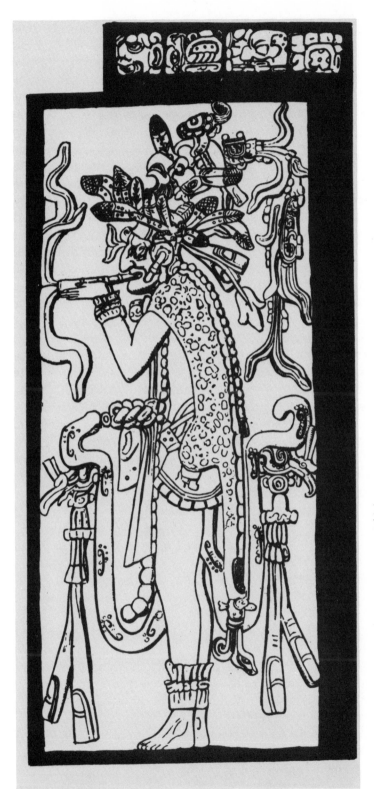

FIG. 27: Jaguar god
blowing smoke to the four winds

Nicotiana tabacum and *N. rustica* are tetraploids, that is to say, they have twice as many chromosomes as expected in the normal complements. Heiser recognizes *N. sylvestris* and *N. octophora* as distinct species that are the likely progenitors of *N. tabacum*, since they are diploids with overlapping distributions in northwestern Argentina. He believes that *N. rustica* arose from *N. paniculata* and *N. undulata* in north central Peru. This domestication is probably as ancient in the New World as maize.

Tobacco consumption by pipe, cigar, and as a snuff was widespread shortly after its introduction into Europe. It was not until the states of western Europe fought the Crimean War that they adopted the habit of cigarette smoking, which has subsequently surpassed all other modes of use in popularity. Not until 1921 did the cigarette in America champion over snuff, cigars, pipes, and chewing tobacco. Cigarettes now usually represent a blend of Turkish and Oriental tobaccos with the milder American tobaccos. The small-leaved Turkish tobaccos are strong and musky in aroma. These blended tobaccos often have such additives as oil of hops, sugar, licorice, glycerine, cider concentrate, coumarin, and rum. Such a list reads like an Indian curry recipe. One peculiar additive comes from St. James Parish in the Mississippi Delta. *Perique* is made by alternately pressing the juice from tobacco leaves and allowing it to be reabsorbed. Over a period of several months a strong black tobacco is produced as a result of this fermentative process that is unlike any other. Of course, the kind of tobacco produced from seed will depend upon soils, climates, curing, and these additives. We must remember that tobacco, like most domesticated plants, also has its varieties. In the manufacture of cigars, Vuelta Abajo, Cuba, produces a cigar that smokers have dubbed unparalleled, while Java and Sumatra produce the finest leaves for use as cigar wrappers.

In Australia, *Duboisia* species under the name *pituri* were the most popular narcotic, but upon the arrival of the English these people became interested in "white fellow *pituri*," that is to say the English smoking and chewing tobaccos from *N. tabacum*. Although some areas of Australia may have used *Nicotiana* species at an earlier time, most accounts trace the use of the native *N. suaveolens*, *N. escelsior*, and *N. gossei* to the adoption of the practices of the English. Fresh flowering stalks, leaves, and even flowers were readily eaten in areas near Ernabella, according to Johnston and Cleland, formerly professors at the University of Adelaide who explored the interior of Australia in the 1930's. Leaves of *N. suaveolens* were dried over hot rocks and chewed into a *bolus* or quid and then rolled in the ashes of the Red Gum tree (*Acacia ligulata*). To hold the sticky mass together, the hair of the wallaby or rabbit was often added. Sticky balls of this tobacco-ash-fur mixture were held between the lips or relegated to the area between the teeth and gums. The *bolus* was alternately chewed and sucked, much as with the leaves of *Erythroxylum coca* in Peru. Like *Duboisia* species, some of these native tobaccos were used by seers for magic and prophecy. As totem plants, they were venerated.

It is rather easy to understand why tobacco has been held in great esteem by aboriginal peoples who have transposed the narcotic effects into their cosmographies and into the psycho-social order as well as the magico-religious rites that involve trance. Thus, among the Mayas the Rain God and the Night God (Jaguar

God) have been portrayed smoking pipes of tobacco (Fig. 27). Among the North American Indians, smoking tobacco was practiced as a peace gesture and was blown to the four winds as a votive offering. Given the present state of information concerning tobacco, it is more difficult to interpret the behavior of Western man in his tobacco addiction. The neural toxins nicotine and nornicotine, which are liquid rather than crystal in their natural state, are as deadly as cyanide. If these toxins were to be isolated from one cigar and administered directly to a human being, he would die almost instantaneously. Neural toxins serve to banish boredom, allay anxiety, and ultimately produce a tranquil stupor. Perhaps tobacco is the best illustration that we have of the inherently irrational nature of man. The smoker is rarely uninformed as to what his fate will likely be as the result of habituation to tobacco. The choice made is a mixture of desire for immediate gratification, existing habituation that would be difficult to break away from, and sometimes an extension of group behavior. Threats of cancer, heart disease, respiratory failure, and birth defects have not changed patterns of smoking significantly; only the targets change. With women's liberation underway, the tobacco industry immediately made women their targets, and the number of women smokers increased dramatically in the United States. Profits to the tobacco industry that well exceed ten billion dollars annually permit extravagant advertising, with a minimum of caution, and permit the legal purchase of influence in the form of governmental lobbyists. It is perplexing to find a society with a deadly national narcotic that is under federal subsidy, hitting hard at persons smoking milder euphoriants that are relatively harmless. We have legislated the death penalty for persons selling *Cannabis* to minors in some states, and at the same time we have supported with tax dollars the tobacco aristocracy that was built in the eighteenth century and persists today. It will present an enigma to the social anthropologist of the future.

HALLUCINOGENS

*"We are such stuff as dreams are made on; and
our little life is rounded with a sleep."*

William Shakespeare, The Tempest
Act IV, Scene 1

OF THE FIVE CLASSES OF DRUGS defined in 1924 by Lewis Lewin, hallucinogens
(psychotomimetics) fall into the intriguing category *phantastica*. The plants in this
group are those that act upon the central nervous system to produce a state in which
there is an alteration of time, consciousness of self, space, and perception of the
physical world. Sensory displacement may accompany a voyage into the realms of
the fantastic and there may be acute sensitivity to color and hearing. Sometimes
these sensations are divided into the categories of auditory, visual, and tactile
hallucinations, but synesthesia may accompany this experience and one sensation
is altered or displaced by another, or the senses become temporarily interchanged. A
perfume becomes red and the sound of a bell in the distance is a vivid blue. The
touch of a piece of silk may produce the sensation of a color comingled with a
fragrance and a most unusual perception of time and place. Polymelia, the sensation
of having many limbs or digits, is not unusual in extreme hallucinations. Past
events may be re-created with an alarming range of detail, and it is possible to
transcend the physical and mundane, even leaving the corporeal body for a period of
soul flight, spirit flight, levitation, or what has been called astral projection. The
world of phantastica is a world in which all things are possible. It is no wonder that
the opulence of late-nineteenth-century French writers such as Theophile Gautier
and Baudelaire has imbued prose and poetry with a peculiar lustre that is ultimately
tied to the world of hallucinogenic plants.

There is an ever-continuing vocabulary that attempts to define the elusive
states characterizing hallucinations; none seems quite satisfactory. We know that
certain plants produce a restricted syndrome of hallucinations such as visual or
audio, while others seem to display their capacities in a pyrotechnic fashion in
which one state merges mercurially into another. By 1932 the French neurobiologist
Raoul Mourgue had analyzed over 7,000 publications on hallucinations in *The
Neurobiology of the Hallucination*, and he concluded that all of the data analyzed
from these sources could not provide him with a theory of hallucinations.
Neurobiologists continue to probe the poorly understood world of the mechanisms

of psychotomimetic plant drugs in an attempt to understand their mode of functioning. The ethnobotanist, on the other hand, seeks to identify the plants capable of producing such profound altered states of consciousness and put them into some meaningful historical context. The ritual use of hallucinations has been the subject of several symposia volumes in the last decade in which an attempt has been made to identify the plant hallucinogens with the myths, rites, and magic that have given them the position of providing shamanic equilibrium, in a psycho-social sense, in diverse cultures. Thus, our understanding is being broadened by a collaboration between chemists, botanists, anthropologists, psychologists, and sociologists. After all, it is a task of the investigator in this realm to attempt to separate the learned psychodrama of a culture from the behavior produced by a plant drug. One of the great collaborations of this century is that of Dr. Richard Evans Schultes of the Harvard Botanical Museum and Dr. Albert Hofmann of the Sandoz Laboratories in Basel, Switzerland. Together these two scientists in 1973 produced the first book to effectively survey *The Botany and Chemistry of Hallucinogens*. It is collaborations such as these that are going to produce a new understanding of a complex subject that has been much misinterpreted.

Geneticists and physiologists are coming closer to an understanding of some of the aspects of the mass of neural circuits called "mind." As with every other function of man, the mind is under chemical control, and there is a chemical basis for the ardor and passion of lust, the subtle sympathies of love, the rage of tyrants, and for "sleep that knits up the ravelled sleeve of care." The use of hallucinogens in an attempt to "expand consciousness" and to probe subconscious states of mind seems an inevitability. A general lack of information has led to an assumption on the part of the public in general that this is the first generation that has had to cope with the complexities of pursuing altered states of consciousness. It is the hope of this author that a historical overview of hallucinogens in world cultures will provide the sort of understanding that may lead to further inquiry rather than judgements. For the moment our lack of precise information on the long-term effects of these psychotomimetics would suggest caution.

It was simpler even a decade ago to state the number of hallucinogens in the Old World versus the New World, but abundant interest in the area of ethnobotany is constantly revealing to us new species of plants in both of these areas that have been used to induce hallucinations. Although it is a consensus that the New World provides substantially more hallucinogens than the Old World, recent investigations into the defunct civilizations in areas such as ancient Assyria, Egypt, and Greece are providing interesting clues into the provoked experience in these ancient civilizations. "The Mysteries" that were those of Eleusis and of temple priests in Babylonia, Mesopotamia, Assyria, and Egypt may be more than the mere ritual and verse that has been invoked by archeologists and anthropologists.

Of the more than 600,000 plant species known to man, about one in ten thousand of those analyzed chemically has revealed a principle that would qualify it as a hallucinogenic plant, but the search goes on. We also are confronted with the dilemma of why certain plants have been historically selected as agents for inducing hallucinations while other plants available to that same culture have been ignored, even though they may have the same potential, and in some instances may have fewer associated toxins.

It is an important observation that unlike the other categories discussed in this book, the true hallucinogens are non-addicting. They may produce the aforementioned disordering of the senses and create a disruption of the ego, but they do not create physiological habituation. I cannot see it as a process without possible hazards, for in probing into the recesses of the mind, in reshaping modes of thought, in repressing the ego and extending experience into undreamed of realms, the individual who is unprepared psychologically may experience a crisis of considerable dimensions. And yet, by contrast, some of these plant drugs have been the most useful adjuncts to therapy in recalcitrant patients who could not otherwise yield to the experiences of psychic extension. In antiquity the shaman was the guide for spirit flight and in some areas of the world he still is. In contemporaneous Western society the physician and the psychotherapist must serve as shaman-guide.

Dr. Alexander Shulgin stated in a symposium on psychotomimetic drugs that sanity is a statistical thing determined by a group of three; it is a minority concept. I find this concept intriguing, for it eliminates "the real world" and relates reality to a society, a time and a place in that society, and a judgement from the majority. Anyone who has used a potent hallucinogen knows that reality becomes a very subjective thing. The paradox is that the intensity of this reality may far exceed the non-provoked reality, or what some might define as a "normal state of being." Perhaps the use of a hallucinogen is a part of the normal, and is a part of being human. Psychotropic means literally to turn the soul or mind, to change the psyche. Is this not a normal human function, and if induced, is it abnormal? Are we not, as Shakespeare tells us, "such stuff as dreams are made on"? Can man endure an unchanging realm of conscious behavior without respite? History would seem to say no.

There is only limited authoritative information on the mode of action of those principles that have been identified as hallucinogenic. In some instances it is thought that the active principle forms a secondary compound in the liver by combining with a protein, in others a hallucinogen is activated by being ammoniated or methylated in the body and exists only as a hallucinogenic precursor before that. In other cases the psychotomimetic is thought to interfere with normal oxidative processes in the brain. Recent efforts indicate the accumulation of materials such as serotonin, normally broken down by the transmission of nerve impulses, that act as a hallucinogenic agent. Some chemicals in this group would seem to break neural synapses or render transmission across them an impossibility. All of these processes are probably extant in different systems, for the chemicals that facilitate such physiological and psychological responses are as diverse as the plants producing them.

In order to systematize the survey of the many hallucinogenic plants of the world, I have thought it best to order them geographically, as an alternative to a chemical ordering or a botanical arrangement would presume too much on the part of the reader. I also believe that this arrangement may be more historically meaningful.

TROPICAL ASIA

A frequent misconception regarding early explorations is that their purpose was to provide spices for European tables; in reality, this trade sought sandalwood, pepper, opium, rhubarb, and aloes not for gourmand palates, but as narcotics, aphrodisiacs, and, most important, medicines. From the ninth to the fifteenth centuries, Venice controlled the trade, having defeated her Genoese competitors. With the fall of Constantinople in 1453, the Portuguese entered the trade and monopolized markets for the next century; during this period the Spaniards sponsored Columbus, who, looking for a trade route to India, stumbled upon America. When in the seventeenth century the Dutch held supremacy of the seas, they initiated ruthless tactics to gain a monopoly of the drug trade. Islands not under Dutch control were plundered for their spices and drug plants, and the few remaining plants were destroyed so that subsequent invaders might not have access to them.

For sixteen years the Dutch entrepreneurs controlled the entire market of nutmeg from Amsterdam. This was a very precious commodity, its seeds being regarded as a medicine of enormous merit. So precious were nutmegs that carved wooden replicas were sold to the ignorant via a black market. Slaves on the ships bringing nutmeg to Europe were castigated for consuming part of the cargo. They knew that a few of the large kernels of the nutmeg seed would relieve their weariness and bring euphoric sensations of an other-worldly nature accompanied by pleasant visions. Nausea and dizziness often followed as the price for this respite from reality, whether the nut was grated and eaten or made into a snuff. The more practical mind of the European saw this seed as a potential medicine and did not hesitate to administer it in the event of severe illness. On that day in February 1685 when the feeble King Charles II was felled by a clot or hemorrhage, one of the numerous unsuccessful attempts to revive him included a decoction of nutmeg. His death a few days later did nothing to detract from the reputation of nutmeg as a very useful drug. Nutmegs encased in silver were worn at night as an inducement to sleep. Aphrodisiacal properties were ascribed to them, and they became a standard element in love potions. In London the rumor spread that a few nuts would act as an abortifacient. A miraculous plant indeed! The ladies who procured abortions were called "nutmeg ladies."

Myristica fragrans is the Latin name for the nutmeg tree, which attains a height of sixty feet and has small, heavy-scented yellow flowers (Pl.17). These dioecious trees are native to the Banda Islands, which were formerly known by the name Nutmeg Islands. It was not until 1512 when the Portuguese reached Banda that nutmeg became known to the Western world. At maturity a pendulous fruit resembling an apricot splits to reveal a dark brown seed about an inch long and covered by a crimson arillus fingering around the seed. The arillus is easily separated from the seed and is known in the spice trade as mace, a delicate condiment. Whole nutmegs minus the seed coats contain fifteen per cent volatile oils; these impart its characteristic flavors.

Hallucinogenic effects from nutmeg were not recorded until 1576, when Lobelius in his *Plantarum seu Stiripium Historia* described a "pregnant English lady who, having eaten ten or twelve nutmegs, became deliriously inebriated." She had undoubtedly heard rumors about the efficacy of nutmeg as an abortifacient: it was fortunate that she did not die from the experience, for a large dose of nutmeg may be lethal. In 1829 the famous biologist Purkinje ate three nutmegs and compared his experience to that of *Cannabis* intoxication (it is interesting to note that this famous biologist was obviously familiar with the effects of *Cannabis* euphoria). Drowsiness seems to accompany the delirium, which may last up to thirty-six hours.

Some doubt has been expressed that nutmeg has ever been a culturally important hallucinogen, but a *Materia Medica* published in Bombay in 1883 indicates that "the Hindus of West India take *Myristica* as an intoxicant." Further evidence derives from an Ayurvedic name for nutmeg, *made shaunda*, which translates as "narcotic fruit." It is well known that nutmeg is mixed with betel nut and snuff in certain parts of southern India. Restrictions against the consumption of hashish in Egypt are reported to have led to the substitution of nutmeg, according to a recent book on poisons. My own observations in Alexandria and Cairo would indicate to me that there is a ready supply of hashish in the streets, and no nutmeg substitution would be necessary. In rural eastern Indonesia, powdered nutmeg is used as a snuff. None of these reports suggests any ritual or religious use for nutmeg. It would seem only a temporal escape. Perhaps the most common use of nutmeg is to be encountered in prisons where other drugs may not be readily available. Some prisons have now dropped nutmeg from their list of kitchen condiments. In most instances it seems to be adopted where the drug of preference is unattainable. The usual side effects include headache, nausea, vertigo, tachycardia, and constipation, making it a less desirable drug than many others.

The response to nutmeg intoxication is extremely diverse. Some individuals experience a profound distortion of time and space and actually have visual hallucinations. These are not so predictable as with hashish, mescaline or LSD. Auditory and tactile hallucinations are not uncommon. Some reports indicate that the participant felt nothing, including the undesirable effects. Perhaps a part of this is predicated on the amount used and the freshness of the material. It is known that nutmeg deprived of its oil fraction has no effects, and nutmeg as purchased in containers in a powdered form is often old and the oils have volatilized or oxidized. Freshly grated nutmeg produces the most profound intoxication. It is the aromatic ethers that seem to be the most likely source of hallucinations. These may be derived from either *Myristica fragrans* or *M. malabarica*.

The mode of action of these aromatic ethers remains obscure. Myristicin constitutes four per cent of the oil of the nut, and twenty-five per cent of this fraction is elemicin, which can be degraded to two potent hallucinogens, TMA (trimethoxy amphetamine) and MMDA (3-methoxy-4, 5-methylenodioxy amphetamine) merely by becoming ammoniated in the body. Crude nutmeg and myristicine (a synthetic) have both been shown to produce a degree of monoamine oxidase inhibition in both in vivo and in vitro testing. Since separate fractions of these aromatic ethers have been tested in human subjects and have shown less effect than a combination of two or more, a synergistic activity has been proposed. In laboratory animals large doses of nutmeg have revealed diseased livers upon autopsy.

In vitro studies have demonstrated the conversion of oil of nutmeg to amphetamines, but as yet it has not been shown to occur in vivo. While the elemicin and myristicin fractions seem the most likely candidates as "pro-hallucinogens," it may be that these two act with another fraction of the oil, perhaps safrol. Safrol is the predominant fraction in the oil of saffron taken from the female parts of *Crocus sativa*. Saffron was used not only as a condiment and a dye, but was regarded as a medicinal narcotic in the ancient Mediterranean and was used in the form of a tea to put unruly children to sleep. If the safrol fraction undergoes demethoxylation, it produces the well-known narcotic MDA (methylenodioxy amphetamine). It has led some chemists to characterize these fractions of nutmeg as the naturally occurring amphetamines, although they are only precursors.

In southeast Asia, especially in cosmopolitan cities such as Bangkok, Thailand, there is a plant product sold as a substitute for opium under the names *mambog* and *kratom*. The plant, *Mitragyna speciosa*, is a member of the coffee family, Rubiaceae. It has a shrubby form, with dichotomous branches terminating in yellow balls of flowers (Pl. 18). *Kratom* is a leafy material that may be smoked like *Cannabis*, and *mambog* is a thick syrup made from the leaves. It is difficult to estimate the antiquity of *kratom* use in tropical Asia, but we do have a report from the year 1895 indicating that the leaves were being sold in the "Straits Settlements" (Malaya) as an opium substitute and as a withdrawal agent. Leaves are either chewed when freshly picked, smoked when dried, or go into the production of *mambog*.

The chemical that acts on both the central nervous system and the sympathetic divisions of the autonomic system has recently been identified as the indole mitragynine. Effects of *kratom* are a pleasant reverie comparable to altered states of consciousness achieved by using hallucinogenic mushrooms such as *Psilocybe* or a small dose of LSD. The chemical skeleton of this organic compound is very similar to the latter. Evidence to date does not indicate that *kratom* is addictive, but it is habit forming. Extended use of *Mitragyna* derivatives results in emaciation, a distended stomach, pallor, darkened lips, dry skin, numbness in peripheral areas, twitching, and anomalous cardiac disorders. Although the primary action on the central nervous system is attributed to mitragynine, which increases the excitability of the medullary portions of the brain, the following eight alkaloids have been isolated may contribute to the characteristic syndrome: ajmalicine, corynan-thedidine, isomitraphylline, mitraphylline, paynantheine, speciophylline, speciofo-line, and speciogynine. The *trans* configuration of mitragynine is of especial interest in that this form of mitragynine is analogous to other psychoactive compounds, such as psilocybin and psilocin from *Psilocybe* mushrooms and lysergic acid amide found in ergot and baby wood rose. In its ability to excite the motor centers of the central nervous system, the preparations of *kratom* and *mambog* suggest cocaine-like functioning. Clearly, this is one of the most complex of the hallucinogens.

TEMPERATE ASIA

In 1972 James H. Sanford of the Department of Religion, University of North Carolina, presented a fascinating account of Japan's "laughing mushrooms" and linked these to some equally curious mushrooms and behavior associated with their consumption in China. His interest began with the reading of a tale of a collection of medieval Japanese folktales. These eleventh-century tales, characterized as folk history, present in Volume Five a story of woodcutters from Kyoto who lost their way in a mountainous region. They encountered in the wilderness a group of four or five Buddhist nuns who were dancing and singing and perceived them to be demons because of their erratic behavior. Upon questioning the women, they were told that these were indeed nuns who had also strayed and, becoming hungry, had roasted and eaten some mushrooms, whereupon they began to laugh and dance about. The woodcutters were both astonished and hungry. The nuns readily shared their mushrooms, and all became giddy, laughing and dancing about together. The mushrooms were called from that time on *maitake* or "dancing mushrooms."

This tale led to Sanford's investigation of possible subsequent accounts of such unusual behavior and the mushrooms causing it. Among other things, he was able to conclude that the tale dated to about A.D. 1000, and the mushrooms were either *Paneolus papilionaceus* or *Pholiota spectabilis* (Figs. 28 & 29). To these he adds the identifications of Imazeki and Hongo, who speak of *waraitake* (the laughing mushrooms) as *Paneolus papilionaceus* and another form of dancing mushroom as *Gymnopilus (Pholiota) spectabilis*. These authors also mention a false "dancing mushroom," *Psilocybe (Stropharia) venenata* or *P. (S.) caerulescens*, since all intoxicate in a similar manner. *Paneolus papilionaceus* was a mushroom identified by Heim as the ingredient being used by witches in Portugal. Furthermore, the same species has been used in the United States for some time for deliberate intoxication; a sort of cheap drunkenness.

Sanford did not terminate his research with the Japanese tale, but read a Chinese work of the Sung period by Yeh Mengte (1077–1148) in which he found a cure for the uncontrollable fits of laughter caused by eating the maple-tree fungus. The cure was eating muddy earth, but more interesting is a Chinese hallucinogen associated with the maple tree and with the sort of laughter reported in the Japanese tale. The Chinese tale was set in the valleys about Mount Ssu-ming in southwestern Cekiang Province, an area closely associated with the T'ien T'ai sect of Buddhism. The mushroom goes unidentified except for its characterization of *chün*. Sanford also located a source for the "laughing fungus" in a work of 1619, which translates as *The Five Fold Miscellany*. This and other later sources seem to add little to the possibility of a deliberate and contextual use of the fungus in either Japan or China. Perhaps this is the lead into an investigation that might provide a relationship between the mushroom and instances of some ritual intoxication.

Cannabis is one of the most ancient hallucinogens of mankind, having been employed by the Chinese over eight thousand years ago (Pls. 19, 20, & 21). Today it enjoys the widest distribution of any of the psychotomimetics and perhaps the

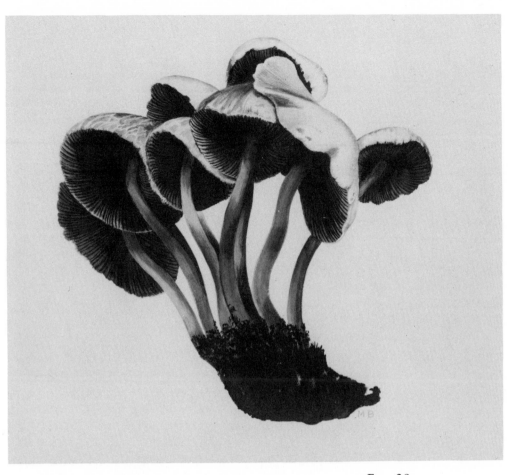

FIG. 28:
Paneolus papilionaceus

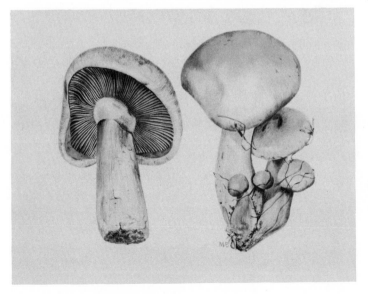

FIG. 29:
Pholiota spectabilis

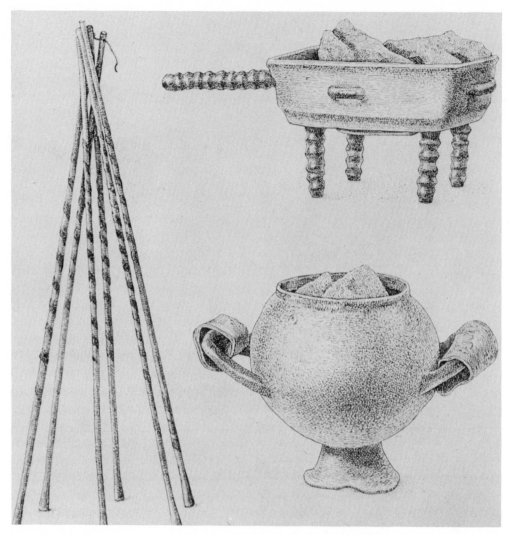

FIG. 30: Scythian *Cannabis* vessels and stakes for vapor tent

widest acceptance in a social, if not legal sense. The ancient Scythians and Assyrians used it to produce an intoxicating smoke that was not burnt in a cigarette, but in a vessel under an animal skin where the intoxicating resins could volatilize and be inhaled (Fig. 30). We have evidence from early Scythian sites as well as the testimony of the historian Herodotus, who referred to the funeral ceremonies of the "howling Scythians." These people built fires and heaped the smouldering coals with *Cannabis* plants which were covered by a sheepskin quilt. Participants would lift the skins and inhale the fumes. The Sanskrit *Zend-Avesta* first mentions this material in 600 B.C. In India the use is as old as soma. Under the name *bhang*, it was one of five sacred plants employed in magical rites to permit freedom from distress and protection from enemies. It was consumed as an intoxicating drink in both

Thrace and India. Galen speaks of "a warm and toxic vapor" produced by eating the seedcakes of *Cannabis*. In the year A.D. 220 we have records of the celebrated Chinese physician and surgeon Hua-T'o performing surgery with *Cannabis* resin in wine.

Hashish, or hasheesh, is the resin obtained from the glandular leaves and floral parts of the female *Cannabis* plant. The term has been derived from the name of a Persian from Hashishin Tus. Al-Hasan ibn-al-Sabbah (A.D. 1124) was tutored in the Batinite tradition and was expected to become a missionary for the sect of Ismailites. A strongly charismatic figure, he drew dissenters from orthodox Moslem thought to his sect of "the New Word" or the Hashishins, from whence we derive the term assassin. It would not be necessary to pursue this history if it were not for the popular belief that Al-Hasan had his followers perform ugly deeds under a *Cannabis* madness. His movement was essentially religiously motivated, and his followers were no more murderous than equally zealous Christians in support of their faith of the new word. Most of the information that we have about Hashishin and his religion comes from descendents of the Mongolian Hulagu, who in 1256 seized the mountain fortress of this cult as well as their fortresses and palaces in Persia and destroyed all books and records of this sect. We do know that this sect was responsible for the founding of hospitals, observatories, and universities. Unfortunately, the name of Hashishin will probably remain associated with murders and *Cannabis*, while his noble deeds are already forgotten.

The word marijuana (marihuana) is derived from the Portuguese *maran guango* and connotes intoxication. Marijuana is perhaps the most popular term for *Cannabis* in the English-speaking world, although synonyms of popular origin in current use now number well over twenty. Sara Bentowa, of the Institute of Anthropological Sciences in Warsaw, has studied the philology and etymology of *Cannabis* from ancient times and compiled over one hundred synonyms for the plant prior to 1936.

There has been considerable controversy over the question of species in the genus, just as botanists of an earlier time debated over the disposition of *Cannabis* into the proper family. While it is now accepted that *Cannabis* is in the family Cannabaceae, it is the contention of a few botanists that there is but a single species in this cosmopolitan genus, that being *C. sativa*. Most taxonomists who have studied the genus recognize at least three species: *C. sativa*, the tall (6–25 feet) plant of northern areas used predominantly for the fiber in its stem; *C. indica*, a low-growing bush of a more southern latitude and high in intoxicating resins; and *C. ruderalis*, a small unbranched invader of other crops in northeastern Europe. This polytypic concept of the genus originated in the eighteenth century with the famous biologist Lamarck and was extended by the Russian botanist Janishevsky in 1924.

The issues surrounding the use and abuse of *Cannabis* are so complex that perhaps the only way in which they might be understood is in terms of historical uses in different areas of the world. In ancient China it was predominantly a medicant for gout, female disorders, rheumatism, malaria, beriberi, constipation, and absentmindedness. As already indicated, it found a place as an anesthesia. Greece had a word for smoking this plant, *cannabeizein*. This often took the form of volatilizing it by placing the resinous top in an incense burner in which myrrh, balsam, and frankincense had been mixed, this in the manner of the shamanic Ashera priestesses of the pre-Reformation temples in Jerusalem, who anointed their skins with the mixture as well. This is possibly the material of the priestess at Delphi.

Democritus (ca. 460 B.C.) knew the plant as *potamaugis*, which was drunk in wine with myrrh to produce delirium and visionary states. Democritus wrote of the immoderate laughter that followed a draught of this decoction. It is of interest to note that Democritus was called "the laughing philosopher." Theophrastus (371–287 B.C.) gave one of the first botanical accounts of the plant under the name *dendromalache*. It was used by the Thracian Getae, a nomadic group, in the sixth century B.C. Their shamans, known as the Kapnobatai, used the smoke to induce visions and oracular trances. Among the Turko-Tartar peoples, shamanic ecstasis played an important role in healing as well as funeral rites, and it has been thought by some that the "howling" reported by Herodotus among the Scythians was characteristic of the shaman or psychopompus. *Cannabis* trances provided the shaman with a spiritual guide to the netherworld.

The Iranian word for this plant was *bangha* and simultaneously referred to mushroom intoxication and *Cannabis* intoxication. Among the ancient Persians, the living as well as the dead could commune with Zarathustra through the intervention of *Cannabis*. From the Iranian tradition the plant found its way to India, where it was not indigenous. It soon became inseparable from religious ceremonies in which it was the "heavenly guide." *Cannabis* intoxication allowed the confused mind to become clarified and the senses to focus on the Eternal. Mixtures of *Cannabis* resin were used before reading holy writ or entering sacred places. This drink called *vijaya* is now often a small amount of resin in milk with various admixtures. The purpose is to attain the celestial union between man and God that cannot be attained in a state of mundane preoccupation. *Vijaya* was the favorite drink of the god Indra, given to man so that he might attain elevated states of consciousness. It seems likely that the route to Africa was by way of India, but it may have been through Saudi Arabia. We know that it was used in the Valley of the Zambezi in pre-Portuguese times (before A.D. 1500). Two uses were preeminent: a smouldering fire was banked with the plants, and the users, prostrate around the fumes, inserted reeds into the smoke and inhaled. The Dervish tradition was to mix *Cannabis* resins with various seed oils and drink the mixture to produce a trance that would provide a revelation. In the Belgian Congo the Balubas were united as brothers-of-*Cannabis* (*bene-Riamba*) when their leader did away with the many different tribal gods of the various territories and provided a union in this wondrous plant. It was smoked in gourds one meter in circumference. In North Africa where *kif* is the name by which the plant is known, it is carried in a pouch of several compartments containing various grades of *Cannabis*. Degrees of esteem or friendship are ascertained by the quality offered. The *kif* room of a house is an essential piece of architecture, for it is in these rooms that oral traditions are passed from generation to generation in a relaxed atmosphere provided by *kif*.

North Europe had a long tradition of using *Cannabis* fibers, whereas the use of the resins is fairly obscure until around 1800. When Napoleon's battered armies returned from the Egyptian campaign, they brought hashish with them. Although the custom of using the resin was not immediately assimilated, it soon became popular in asylums for quieting unruly mental patients. It was, about mid-century, taken up by a group of writers and artists who founded *Le Club des Haschischins*. This elitist group met in the elegant Hotel Pinodan on the fashionable Ile St. Louis in an atmosphere of chimerical phantasmagoria that would lend itself to hallucinatory experiences. Dr. Moreau, who in 1841 began to treat the mentally ill with hashish (with great success), was the primary officiant at the monthly meetings. From a crystal vase he would dispense a spoonful of green hashish paste, pronouncing the dictum, "This will be deducted from your share in paradise." These monthly meetings were held regularly and conducted with the formality of a religious service. The intoxication that followed had many manifestations, but as Baudelaire pointed out, it would be within the confines of a man's physical and moral temperament, "Hashish will be for a man's familiar thoughts and impressions, a mirror that exaggerates, but always a mirror." It is the ceremonial aspect of this practice that makes it so very interesting. Is an elitist group of intellectuals sharing their ecstasies really so far removed from the shared ritual of the "howling Scythians"?

In 1963 the Mexican ethnologist Roberto Williams Garcia published a paper on *Cannabis* as "santa rosa" or "the herb which makes one speak." Among the Tepecanos in northwest Mexico, it was reported by Lumholtz in 1902 that *Cannabis sativa* was used under the name "rosa maria" when peyote was not available. Likewise, the Tepehua living in the mountains of Vera Cruz, Hidalgo, and Puebla use the "santa rosa" in a ceremony that is as elaborate as any religious activity that may be imagined. Prayers, music, rhythmic movement, dancing, and whistling all figure into this service in which *Cannabis* intercedes with the Virgin Mary as an earth deity. It is thought to be alive and is equated with the sacred heart of Jesus, which is displayed on an alter where the herb is sanctified. Were it not for the ritual use and praying, it is believed that the plant could steal a man's soul and make him sick, perhaps even kill him. It might produce a "fleeting madness" that could only be controlled by a shaman. If venerated and used sacramentally, however, it cures and intercedes for the sinner.

In conjunction with the above, it is interesting to note the sacramental aspects of the plant's growth in montane Oaxaca. Here we find as much ritual as in the use of the plant as a sacrament. The high altitude and volcanic soils produce a particularly potent strain of *Cannabis*. The intense ultraviolet light may be responsible for converting some of the inert cannabinoids to the active delta-one isomeric form. Agricultural traditions here are ancient, and we have no date for the advent of *Cannabis*. It has been suggested that it is post-conquest in this area, but that is by no means a certainty. *Cannabis* does not flourish in such extremes of climatic and edaphic pressures, rather it grows in a "tortured" fashion. This is further exaggerated by severe pruning and by pinching out the young shoots to form the plant into an urn shape. In establishing this form the resins containing the potent cannabinoids volatilize and recondense within the confines of the plant form until it is encrusted with the narcotic material. This brings about hormonal changes in the plants that turn them to a bright red to red-purple. The plant looks like anything but *Cannabis*. As the blood-like color begins to appear, and the plant shimmers with crystalline resins, it is "crucified" by having two wooden splinters driven through the basal stem in the manner of a cross. The association between this practice and the aforementioned association between the plant and Christ is hardly fortuitous. These syncretic Christo-pagan religious traditions are suggested by the urn-shaped "heart" of red, the crystals that shimmer like traditional shamanic rock crystals, and the ritual crucifixion after which the plant is pulled from the ground and hung upside down. Even if the Indian is at this time concerned primarily with the potency of the resins, the religious implications are inescapable. This does not constitute the hashish that is exported, but an indigenous sacramental material.

There was a time when the resins of *Cannabis*, in a tincture, were a valuable medicine easily obtained in any drugstore. As recently as 1930, it was legal to utilize *Cannabis* and its derivatives in all but sixteen states, but the Tax Act of 1937 implemented such rigid controls that it was effectively eliminated from most pharmacies. The Federal Bureau of Narcotics was established in 1930 and yet little was done between 1930 and 1937, and it seems that marijuana was not considered a problem of any consequence. The era of prohibition of alcohol was in full swing. The Treasury Department reported in 1931 that "publicity tends to magnify the extent of the evil." Shortly thereafter the repeal of prohibition laws led to a greater interest in eliminating marijuana. By 1936 there was no indication that patterns of *Cannabis* use were changing, but priorities had shifted and the Federal Bureau of Narcotics spoke of "the urgent need for vigorous enforcement of cannabis laws," and with this they initiated the infamous "educational campaign" in which the plant was suddenly dubbed "the killer weed" that induced "reefer madness." Newspapers also changed their priorities, and the stories fed to them of mass murders, rape, and insanity were published widely and often repeated as evidence of the enormous danger. Posters were distributed to schools, and anonymously authored films depicted lives ruined by *Cannabis*.

One bit of irony is that in the formulation of laws by various states against *Cannabis* it is evident that many of the legislators were unsure of the plant that they were prohibiting. These laws were enacted in addition to the Uniform States Laws Conference of 1932. Thus, *Cannabis* can be found as "locoweed," "peyote," and even as "mushrooms." Most states prohibited marijuana under the Uniform Narcotic Drug Act along with opiates and made the penalties commensurate with opium use. Ironically, marijuana is not considered a narcotic under federal law, but as late as 1960 Commissioner Harry Anslinger gave testimony before the House of Representatives that marijuana use led to a "sort of jaded appetite." He mentioned New York and Los Angeles as being the centers of the problem and stated, "They start on marijuana and . . . well, they switch to heroin."

By 1962 the White House Conference on Narcotic and Drug Abuse heard testimony from senators and judges who resented harsh and unrealistic penalties and the extreme injustice of the existing laws. By 1967 the President's Commission on Law Enforcement and Administration of Justice suggested that the hazards of marijuana were exaggerated and that long criminal sentences were unjust. It became apparent that the legislation was more harmful to society in its enforcement than the problem it was designed to control. If the average taxpayer was provided with an inventory of court costs and criminal maintenance costs, there would be a national scandal of unprecedented proportions.

Through a process of slow but steady repeal, old laws are gradually being supplanted with laws that tolerate a modicum of marijuana as a slight offense, usually a misdemeanor that is subject to a small fine or overlooked. There is no evidence that in those states where the laws pertaining to *Cannabis* have been relaxed there is any increase in criminal behavior. All evidence is to the contrary. This country is finally learning that severe punitive measures have never deterred a populace from indulging in those things that they enjoy. As the old propaganda is fading, respectable institutions and researchers are investigating the real physiological effects of regularly using *Cannabis*. A really thorough report has yet to be issued. Some hazards, such as lowered testosterone levels, seem to be established. The entire picture has yet to come in.

The attempt to regulate large-scale sale and transit of *Cannabis* by dusting the plants by plane with herbicides such as Paraquat has led to the dangers associated with herbicide consumption, for the suppliers still harvest the poisoned plants and market them without warning. The United States government has to face the embarrassment of a scandal whose effects far overreach the use of marijuana. We will have to see what long-term effects might be wrought by herbicides that have in some instances shown to be carcinogenic.

The resins of *Cannabis* have been given to dogs in massive doses without a single fatality. Whether smoked or ingested, the usual effect is a euphoric, non-aggressive feeling often accompanied by an increased appetite. As it is usually smoked, the effect lasts for about two hours. When ingested, the euphoria may be prolonged up to twelve or more hours. This depends upon the quality of the resin or leafy material: that is to say, the amount of delta-1-tetrahydrocannabinol present, as it is the primary euphoriant. When d-1-THC was administered intravenously in experiments carried out under the auspices of the National Institute of Mental Health, it was found this component persists in the blood plasma for more than three days, after which it is completely metabolized. The metabolites leave the body in urine and feces after eight days. However, THC, as a non-polar compound, is lipophilic and accumulates in fatty tissues of the body. This may explain the phenomenon of "reverse tolerance" in which chronic users need progressively *less* of the drug to feel the effects. Naive smokers are often disappointed in the failure to feel any significant effects. This data stands in marked contrast to the ever-increasing need for larger doses of such drugs as heroin and nicotine.

The specific role of delta-1-THC is to affect the central nervous system by altering the turnover rates of such neurotransmitters as norepinephrine, serotonin, and acetylcholine. The negative effects are predominantly *potential* hazards at this point. The reduction in testosterone and deleterious effects on the bronchial system are established. The conjectural hazards that are under investigation are possible chromosomal damage, interference with the immune system, interference with DNA synthessis, irreversible brain damage, marked personality changes. These are all under investigation as *suspected* rather than known effects. If we enumerate the hazards of alcohol and cigarette tobacco on human health, it is clear that both present a greater number of known health and social hazards than *Cannabis*. It should be noted that studies conducted in Jamaica of users who had been chronically involved with heavy *Cannabis* use for over nineteen years failed to produce evidence of the above suspected effects. Further, no organic or physiological addiction develops, and withdrawal symptoms are not evident. As with most drugs, psychic dependence and habituation may follow protracted use. The experience of true hallucinations is dependent upon the utilization of very intoxicating forms of hashish in substantial amounts.

Soma is known to most readers as the stimulant, euphoriant and hallucinogen in Aldous Huxley's novel *Brave New World*. Few people know that the plant soma actually exists and has been used as a narcotic since the time of India's earliest civilizations. In Ancient Indian mythology Soma, the brother of Indra, was the giver of health, courage, long life, a sense of immortality, and almost every other virtue known. As a narcotic, soma is thought to have originated in the Hindu Kush mountain range of northeast Afghanistan. There is evidence that Aryan invaders carried the plant to India and Persia, where it was readily adopted because of its psychoactive properties. Many of the hymns of the *Rig-Veda*, which were sung earlier than 800 B.C., refer to soma as a liquor and as a god. Recent accounts of the history of *Cannabis* have attempted to equate hashish with soma or homa. Homa is a plant derivative celebrated by Zarathustra, prophet to the ancient Iranians. There is every reason to believe that these are the same plants, but it is unlikely that either is *Cannabis* or a preparation of hashish. In *Rig-Veda* IX 113, soma is spoken of as a fragrant liquor, and in *Rig-Veda* X 85:3 there is a description of soma drinkers who "crush the juice from the plant." Neither of these suggests hashish or its mode of preparation. Phillipe de Felice, who wrote extensively on the uses of drugs in religion, adduced evidence that soma was a creeper or a vine, and *Cannabis* is bushy or upright.

Attempting to establish the identity of soma in over 144 hymns of the *Rig-Veda* has occupied ethnobotanists for some considerable time. These writings of the earliest settlers in the Indus basin are deliberately elusive on the point of the identity of soma. In this area and Iran there are several plants that are used under the name soma or homa, and yet these may not represent the soma of antiquity. The sporadic references to the plant in the *Rig-Veda* are elliptical and even contra-dictory. This plant that makes the gods dance and rejoice, produces mental exhilaration, increases the greatness of the priest in his sanctuary and of men, is strong drink for the omnipotent, is expressed by pounding it from the plant with stones, is mixed with milk, it speaks from the wooden bowl, it has swollen stalks which are milked like udders. These are a few of the most direct allusions to soma; others are far more oblique. We are also faced with the dilemma of distinguishing between references to Soma, the god, and soma as a plant or plant product. Although most of these are concentrated in Mandala IX of the *Rig-Veda*, they may be found throughout the work. One major obstacle to uncovering the plant soma is the disagreement between Vedic scholars as to the precise interpretation of these texts. Max Muller, one of the greatest of Vedic scholars, stated in the preface to his 1891 translation of this work that translators of Vedic mandalas "ought to be decipherers, and that they are bound to justify every word of their translation in exactly the same manner in which the decipherers of hieroglyphic or cuneiform inscriptions justify every step they take." In the continuing Vedic scholarship this dictum has not always been followed, and literal interpretation has too often given way to poetic license and interpretation over translation. This is true of the translations of Wilson and Cowell, Griffith and Langlois.

The most recent assay to identify soma has been attempted by R. Gordon Wasson. Wasson relied on the translation of Geldner and that of Renou. It is the most thorough attempt yet to answer the age-old question of the botanical identity of soma, and it was done with the authoritative aid of W. D. O'Flaherty, an expert on Vedic culture and linguistics. Wasson perceived in these texts the absence of any mention of roots, leaves, branches, seeds, or fruits, and since the authors of the *Rig-Veda* do not mention these components, Wasson believes that they did not exist. Therefore, he asserts, the plant must have been a mushroom. Since the fly agaric, *Amanita muscaria*, is a montane plant and has a history of serving as an intoxicant among Siberians, it is put forth as the soma of the Hindu Kush or Himalaya foothills (Pl. 22). Wasson is aware of the limitations imposed by the infrequent presence of substantial numbers of these plants in the areas identified. This he believes may be answered by the assertion that Vedic priests had porters traveling to the forest belts of Eurasia to supply "the Divine Plant." This journey of thousands of miles to procure a plant considered divine hardly seems likely. It is difficult to find a single instance of an ancient culture that culled its sacred narcotic plants from a distant source. Some contenders for soma from previous investigators have been *Periploca aphylla*, *Ephedra* spp., *Rheum* sp., and *Sarcostemma brevistigma* (Pls. 23 & 24). Before dismissing these plants from the list of possibilities, we must investigate some of the assertions in light of their probability. As D. H. Ingalls, a Vedic scholar and supporter of Wasson's thesis, states, "Not all the epithets remarked on by Wasson need to be taken just as he takes them." Ingalls further notes, "I think Wasson's basic identification is a valuable discovery. But when a new tool is given to scholars, it is as important to prevent its misapplication as it is to recognize its value." He goes on to discount the Wasson thesis of "the third sieve," which states that the worshippers drank soma pissed out of the bodies of the priests. The interpretation is limited to a single verse in ten thousand verses of the *Rig-Veda* and is an extension of a practice among Siberians unknown to ancient Vedic people.

A few years ago a German pharmacologist, Hummel, wrote a treatise on soma in which he identified the plant as *Rheum palmatum*, or one of several other Asiatic species of rhubarb. The inherent problem is that *Rheum* species are non-narcotic. He suggested that any of four species of rhubarb were crushed and fermented with sugar or honey to give an intoxicating beverage. Max Muller instigated the idea of soma being a fermented beverage based upon the two kinds of intoxication mentioned in the *Rig-Veda*: that of soma was without "evil effect" and that of beer was said to produce anger and folly. Each type of intoxication is based upon a different word. This has led to the supposition that soma could not be an alcoholic beverage. We need only look into the Christian tradition to find wine as a sacrament representing the blood of Christ, and wine as a mocker. Such a duality should not so easily disconcert translators. One of the attributes in these Sanskrit texts is that of intoxication and another is sweetness. Rhubarb leaves are emetic, and we might suggest that ritual emesis has been almost universally known as an act of cleansing and purification.

About the time of Hummel's thesis, a theory was advanced by the pharmacologist Quazilbash that soma was either *Ephedra pachyclada* or *E. intermedia*. Both are natives to the mountains of northwest India and have the advantage of being leafless, thus more in accord with the Vedic descriptions than *Rheum*, which has a very large leaf. Quazilbash maintains that in order to fit these Vedic hymns the plant had to be soaked in milk, crushed, filtered, mixed with honey, and the brew allowed to ferment. Such a mixture would then contain alcohol as well as ephedrine and pseudoephedrine and would serve as a psychoactive plant that would produce not only the stupor of alcohol, but the "exhilaration" that the *Rig-Veda* speaks of repeatedly. It seems clear that alcohol alone could serve only as a neural depressant and could not account for the states of ecstasy that soma provides. Even today these leafless, sun-loving plants are prepared in Khyber and parts of Afghanistan by boiling them in milk. The brew is thought to be an aphrodisiac and is most certainly a stimulant. Could this be a vestigial practice relating to an earlier soma ceremony? It is not an untenable hypothesis.

Those who have proposed *Sarcostemma viminale* (*Asclepias viminale*) as the holy herb fail to take into account that it is African and not Asian, and the juice is quite toxic, finding use as a fish poison. If we consider which plants found in Pakistan and the Hindu Kush and Pamir mountains of northwest India might be likely candidates, two come to mind: *Periploca aphylla*, a leafless decumbent herb or liana with milky latex, or the related *Periploca hydaspidis*. It was in 1885 that Julius Eggeling, noted for his Sanskrit translations, proposed *Sarcostemma acidum* as soma. Eggeling expressed doubts over his assertion, but indicated that every possibility seemed to favor *Sarcostemma brevistigma* (*S. acidum*). This leafless sprawling plant has many of the attributes found in the *Rig-Veda*. It is a series of branching stems that are quite leafless, and it grows in full sun (IX:86). When the seeds are released from the capsule, they emerge through a single suture that is like the opening of an eye (IX:10 and 97). These seeds, typical of the family, are released in a cloud of silvery comose down after leaving the leathery fruit coat, "he abandons his envelope . . . with what floats he makes continually his vesture of grand-occasion" (IX:71), and soma "shines together with the sun" (IX:2); "he has taken the back of heaven to clothe himself in a spread-cloth like to a cloud" (IX:69). We could give further examples in which the comose down is a cloud or silver or like sheep. The copious milky juice of *Sarcostemma* is reflected in these verses of the *Rig-Veda*: "When the swollen stalks were milked like cows with udders" (VIII:9), "Milking the dear sweetness from the divine udder . . ." (IX:107), "The udder of the cow is swollen; the wise juice is imbued with its streams" (IX:93). These allusions are extremely frequent. As to the "navel of the earth" (IX:72), we have the perfect figuring of a navel in the round involuted center of the flower of *Sarcostemma*. It is this that gives way to the leathery fruit—"The hide is of bull, the dress is of sheep" (IX:70)—that conceals the seed with attached comose down. The form of this fruit is not unlike the horns of steers or bulls, "This bull, heaven's head . . ." (IX:27). Thus, we present but a few of the many verses in the *Rig-Veda* that could be applied to *Sarcostemma acidum*. Wasson has found them equally applicable to *Amanita muscaria*, the mushroom.

We know that *Sarcostemma brevistigma* is used in India today under the name soma, as are several other plants including *Ephedra* species. It may be that all of these are surrogates, or it is quite possible that *Sarcostemma brevistigma* is the plant soma of antiquity. A thorough chemical analysis of the latter to establish the presence of an intoxicating narcotic is in order. It is known that the dried stem is an emetic in Indian medicine, but what of the fresh milky latex? Certainly the herb is worthy of more investigation than has been conducted to date. In a volume entitled *Medicinal, Economic, and Useful Plants of India* by Sudhir Kumar Das, the foreword notes that the "therapeutic uses of plant materials have been quoted from records of the findings made through the ages by Hindoo Ayurvedic Pharmacists." In this compendium of ancient sources, *Sarcostemma brevistigma* is listed with the following note: "Herb. Plant juice is *intoxicating* and blood purifying." Such evidence is only circumstantial, but most intriguing. We must keep in mind that soma was a dangerous drug, that on occasion made Indra, brother of Soma, quite sick.

The contention by Wasson that soma is irrefutably and without a doubt the basidiomycete *Amanita muscaria* is disconcerting. No one has done a more thorough study than Wasson in an attempt to identify the plant soma, and his assertions must carry the weight that is commensurate with the scholarship that is to be found in *Soma, Divine Mushroom of Immortality*. The reader must bear in mind that interpretation is a thing apart from translation, and the ideal interpretation would come from a Vedic scholar who is also a botanist. Wasson's scholarship has opened new doors for us and is not to be taken lightly. It is a model for ethnobotanical research. Whether this resolves the age-old question of soma must be left to the reader.

What is the history behind the fly agaric, *Amanita muscaria*, that might engender a thesis such as that advanced by Wasson? We know that this mushroom contains the toxin muscarine in varying amounts, depending upon the area in which the fungus grows. It also contains the hallucinogens ibotenic acid and muscimole. This mushroom may be found in the temperate areas of the world following the belts of birches, beeches, alders, and pines. In its more southerly distribution it may be found about groves of eucalyptus and oaks. In the histories of the north European countries it appears as the mushroom in children's books having a red cap flecked with white. It is almost always portrayed in stories involving elves and dwarfs, the mystical little people of the forest found in the legends of most north temperate cultures. It was Lewis Carroll (Charles L. Dodgson) who popularized the idea that a mushroom could make a person very large or very small in the eyes of those who partake of it. He had read a review of Cooke's manual on British fungi that contained an account of the properties of *Amanita muscaria;* these were translated into the experiences of Alice when she encountered a prophetic caterpillar in Wonderland.

We know of the antiquity of *Amanita muscaria* intoxication among the tribes of northeastern Asia, the Tungus, Yakuts, Chukches (Chukchees), Koryaks, and Kamchadales. It has also been used extensively among the Finno-Ugrian peoples, the Ostyak and Vogul. The earliest account of these practices was narrated to Europeans when in 1730 a Swedish army officer published his account of imprisonment in Siberia. In 1762 Oliver Goldsmith described his experiences of the use and ritual surrounding this colorful fungus. Since the mushroom is not abundant in northeast Asia, a curious practice has developed. Women of a tribe chew the dried fungus into a pulp, which is rolled into sausage-shaped pieces of a few inches in length. These are eaten by the men of the tribe. Two fungi are usually enough to produce a state of gaiety and exuberance. After passing through the kidneys, the mushroom is detoxified of muscarine and yet the potent muscimole, produced by the decomposition of ibotenic acid, is still abundant in the urine. As testimony to this, we have the words of Goldsmith:

> The poorer [Tartars] post themselves around the huts of the rich and watch [for] the opportunity of the ladies and gentlemen as they come down to pass their liquor, and holding a wooden bowl catch the delicious fluid. Of this they drink with the utmost satisfaction and thus they get as drunk and as jovial as their betters.

Keenan, who was among the Chukches in 1870, reported that a single mushroom was sufficient to keep a band intoxicated for a week, and a single mushroom would fetch three or four reindeer. This is interesting in light of experiments with *Amanita muscaria* in Cambria Pines, California. My informant relayed to me an experience in which he consumed eight of these fungi. Only after such a large dose did he feel any effects, and these were loss of motor coordination, paranoia, and uncontrolled speech. Obviously this fungus shows great variability throughout its range. The other possibility is that an in vivo processing of ibotenic acid to muscimole may be more efficient in bodies of differing physiology. If ibotenic acid decarboxylates and loses water, it becomes five times as potent, for it is then changed to muscimole. Muscazone is found in lesser amount and is pharmacologically less active.

Could this Siberian tradition be allied to the cult of soma? Could this area have been one of the sources for *Amanita muscaria* via an incredibly long trade route? Is this the source for the practice of the priest pissing soma as indicated in the *Rig-Veda* interpreted by Wasson? We know that the Siberian uses involved eating the mushroom after it had been dried in the sun or over a fire, extracting the juices in water and sometimes drinking them with an admixture of reindeer milk. These practices do correspond to many of those indicated in verses of the *Rig-Veda.* The practice of mixing the mushroom with the juice of *Vaccinium uliginosum* or

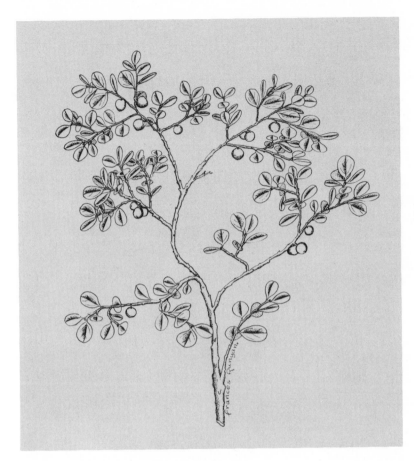

F<small>IG.</small> 31:
Vaccinium uliginosum

Epilobium angustifolium is most interesting (Figs. 31 & 32). In Millspaugh's *American Medicinal Plants*, he mentions several species of *Epilobium* as being used for cramps, diarrhoea, and dysentery. The preparation involves chopping and pounding the entire plant. In addition to the expected effects, he noted that the tincture "caused some symptoms that must have been due to so large a drink . . . symptoms that we are prone to lay to the alcohol." Citing the works of Dr. Wright, who took one-half ounce of the tincture and became intoxicated, we have reason to believe that perhaps there is an intoxicating principle in *Epilobium*, for one-half ounce of a tincture of the plant plus alcohol is a small amount of alcohol in terms of giddiness or intoxication. This same author says of *Vaccinium uliginosum* that it is intoxicating and narcotic. Could it be that some of the effects ascribed to the *berserker* of Scandinavia, who went into impassioned frenetic states of orgies and murder, used not only *Amanita muscaria*, but also these narcotic admixtures? *Vaccinium vitis* was used by the Shakers as a substitute for the related *Arctostaph-ylos uva-ursi*, whose leaves were smoked as *sagack-homi* in Canada and as *kinikinik* among western hunters. These admixtures to the mushroom are much ignored.

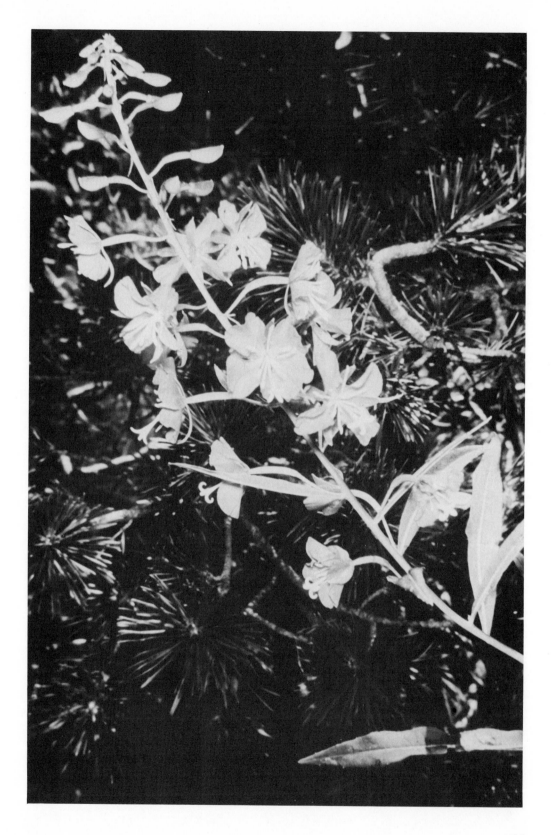

John Allegro, who has distinguished himself as a translator of ancient languages, extended the *Amanita* argument in a book entitled *The Sacred Mushroom and the Cross*. Using linguistic arguments that begin with Sumerian tablets from Arcad and Erech, he traces the mushroom through several cultures and finds it to be a focal point in the Christian tradition. The strong sexual interpretations of these practices all but occlude the argument. One strong point in favor of Allegro's argument is a fresco dating from 1291 on a wall of a deserted church in Plaincourault (Indre, France) which shows Adam and Eve posed on either side of the "Tree of Life" depicted as a large branched *Amanita muscaria* with a serpent wrapped about it. The forbidden fruit in the mouth of the serpent, Satan, is either an apple or a piece of the red *Amanita* cap (Pl. 25). Did the celebration of *Amanita* as a sacred plant exceed that of all psychotropics from many different cultures? Did this tradition originate in the cult of soma among the Vedic peoples? Was soma really *Amanita*, or *Ephedra*, or *Sarcostemma*? One thing remains a certainty: the story of soma has not yet reached its terminus, and the ancient scribe who once penned the following characters in Sanskrit had a yet unraveled secret:

> *Heaven above does not equal one half of me.*
> > *Have I been drinking soma?*
> *In my glory I have passed beyond earth and sky.*
> > *Have I been drinking soma?*
> *I will pick up the earth and place it here or there.*
> > *Have I been drinking soma?*
>
> Rig-Veda X:119, 7–9

Datura is a genus of almost pan-temperate and pan-tropical distribution, and the origin of this highly variable genus is disputed by botanists. The narcotic qualities of *Datura* led to its use as a medicine and mind-altering agent at a very early date in both the Old and the New worlds. Avicenna, the Arabian physician of the eleventh century, noted the intoxication produced by a small amount of the *Datura* "nut" (seed) and wrote of its value in medicine. The generic epithet was derived from early Arabic names for *Datura*: *datora* and *tatorah*. Both of these may be traced to the term *dutra* in India or some of the early Sanskrit writings, in which it is mentioned as *dhustura* and *unmata*. These were probably all names for a single species, *Datura metel* (Fig. 33). The specific epithet of *metel* may derive from the Arabic drug of which Avicenna wrote, *jouz-mathel*. While it is thought that the greatest area of ritual use is now in the area from north Mexico through South America, I believe that this may be due to our lack of knowledge of some of the earliest practices in the Old World, where the plant dates to prehistory. Perhaps no more diverse kinds of practices exist with respect to hallucinogenic plants than we find in *Datura* intoxication. This may seem astonishing considering the extremely toxic nature of the entire plant. It is equally curious that the customs surrounding

FIG. 32: *Epilobium angustifolium*

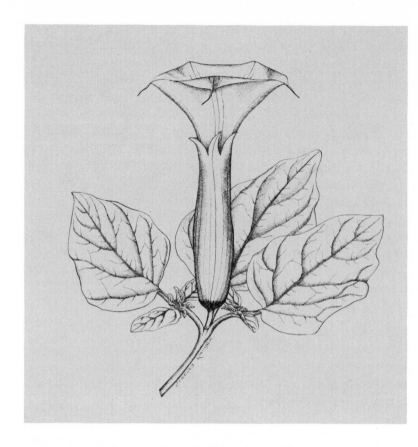

FIG. 33:
Datura metel

the use of *Datura* in temperate Asia at a very early date parallel those of contemporary native peoples of the New World.

Because a concoction of ground seed with water has the power to stupefy, it became a popular drug among thieves and criminals who would use this drug, often with hashish added, to intoxicate their victims. This was a common practice in India, where the same plant was used to treat over twenty diseases including pneumonia, heart disease, mumps, sexual perversions, toothworm, hysteria, epilepsy, and other real or imagined conditions. The liquid extracts of *Datura metel* were useful in drugging young girls and exploiting them as prostitutes; subsequently they would employ extracts of the herb as "knockout drops" to take advantage of their clients. It is no wonder that in India the plant came to have an evil reputation, and those who used it were the *dhatureas*. Only in China was it without the reputation of an evil plant, for there it was sacred and received droplets of water when Buddha spoke. It originated when Buddha promulgated the law. It was then that the plants descended from heaven. Both the flowers and seed of *Datura alba* were used in China under the name *man-t'o-lo* for pustules, swollen feet, prolapsus ani, colds, cholera, and a host of nervous disorders. Equal quantities of this plant and *Cannabis*, dried, pulverized, and steeped in wine, were used to perform operations and cauterizations without pain. It was noted that when used as a medicant *D. alba* often produced a giddy state of laughing and dancing. We do not have a fine record of magico-religious use as we do in the Americas.

SOUTH PACIFIC

Kaempferia galanga is an attractive herbaceous perennial found in loamy soils and shaded areas of New Guinea, India, Malaya, the Moluccas, and the Philippines (Pl. 26). From a pair of glossy deep green leaves there emerges a spike bearing a few pale white flowers mottled violet and having a creamy yellow throat. Under the name *gisól*, the rhizome is used as a ginger-like condiment, and the juices are expressed for sore throats, to accelerate scar tissue formation, and on boils and similar skin eruptions. A related species of tropical Asia, *K. angustifolia*, figures importantly in cough medicines. Because of the fragrance of the rhizome, it is also important in perfumes. In Cambodia, *K. pandurata* is used in colic and stomach ailments, and in Java and surrounding territories the species *K. rotunda* can be found in materia medica as being official for gastric complaints. It is said that *gisól* is useful in severe headache and relieves pain at childbirth. Apart from these fascinating medical applications for this plant, it has been regarded by some groups in New Guinea as a hallucinogen. As *maraba*, the oily juice of the rhizome is consumed. Thus far it has not been possible to identify a psychoactive principle from *K. galanga* or any related species, and we might suspect it to be a semi-sacred plant around which an elaborate psychodrama mimicking hallucinations is witnessed; however, there are a number of plants that have been demonstrated to be psychoactive for which we have no phytochemical information that would support these as hallucinogens. This is the only member of the ginger family that has been reported as a hallucinogen.

Agara is the name by which the Papuans know the timber tree *Galbulmima (Himantandra) belgraveana* (Fig. 34). This is one of the several species found growing in eastern Australia and eastern Malaysia. A decoction of both the leaves and bark is made and added to leaves from *Homalomena ereriba*, an herbaceous aroid (Fig. 35). The resulting mixture, when drunk, or the bark and leaves chewed together, produces fits of violent intoxication accompanied by spectacular visions and dream-like states that terminate in a deep somnolence. Reports from the Papua, New Guinea, Scientific Society indicate that several isoquinoline alkaloids have been isolated from *Galbulmima belgraveana*, among these himbosine, himbacine, himgaline and others. The structure of most of these alkaloids has now been identified, but none seems to show any hallucinogenic activity. Only himbacine's anti-spasmodic action would seem to make it more suspect than the others. While no hallucinogenic compounds have been isolated from *Homalomena ereriba*, *H. rubescens* of Malaysia is used as a fish poison under the name *ipoh*. Chemical studies of the *Homalomena* species are few, and yet over one hundred forty species are known from tropical Asia and South America.

The islands of Hawaii are famous for the attractive plant materials shipped to the mainland of the United States and to the rest of the world to be used in dried flower arrangements or as seeds in jewelry. Prominent among these is the "Hawaiian baby wood rose," which is not a member of the rose family, but is a tropical woody liana of the morning glory family (Convovulaceae). The black seeds within the capsule, which forms after the appearance of the flower, have been used among the poorer Hawaiians for a "high." Unfortunately, the complex alkaloids of these seeds of *Argyreia nervosa* provide not only hallucinations, but a hangover characterized by blurred vision, vertigo, and physical inertia (Fig. 36). In the genus *Argyreia* there are thirteen species containing amides of lysergic acid *(speciosa, nervosa, acuta, barnesii, wallichii, capitata, splendens, osyrensis, aggregata, hainanensis, obtusifolia,* and *pseudorubicunda)*. It was not until 1963 that the presence of amides of lysergic acid were ascertained to be present in *Argyreia* species. Since then there have been several embargos, and a great deal of controversy over the propriety of shipping these fruit capsules and seeds throughout the world. The presence of D-lysergic acid (ergine), isoergine, chanoclavine, elymoclavine, and ergonovine are responsible for the effects experienced, but it is the D-lysergic acid that is responsible for the potent hallucinatory experience. Species of *Ipomoea, Rivea, Claviceps,* and *Stictocardia* are all chemically related to *Argyreia* and will be discussed in the context of their geographical origins and places where they are used. Suffice it to say that all of these are the natural sources for chemicals that are closest to the most potent psychotomimetic known, LSD-25, and most have an antiquity of use extending over hundreds of years.

One of the most fascinating recent ethnobotanical studies covering the area of New Guinea was presented by Harold Nelson at the sixty-ninth Annual Meeting of

Fig. 34: *Galbulmima belgraveana*   Fig. 35: *Homalomena* cf. *ereriba*

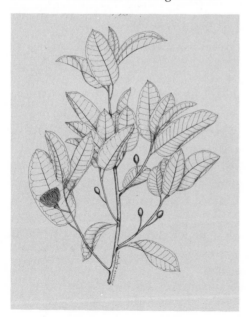
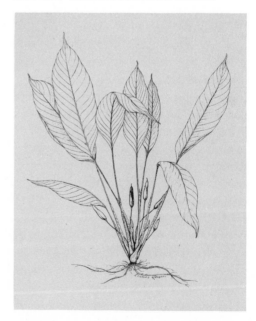

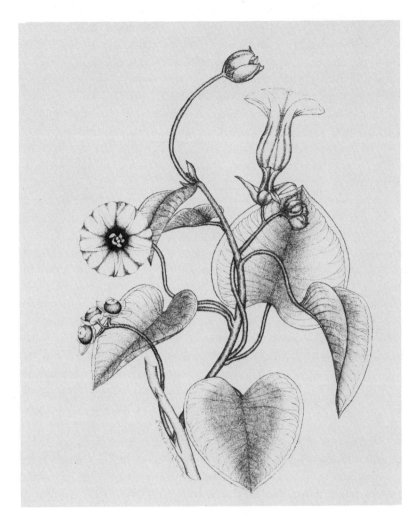

Fig. 36:
Argyreia nervosa

the American Anthropological Association in November 1970. "Mushroom madness" had been laconically noted by Fr. William Ross in 1936, and an inquiry into this phenomenon was initiated by Marie Reay, who worked in the Wahgi Valley in the Western Highlands of New Guinea. Nelson lived with the Kaimbi people in the Bebilyer Valley along the southern slopes of the Kubors during 1967–68 and documented some of the lore associated with this curious seasonal madness. These people know the mushrooms of the area as *nonda*, and the effects of tremors, multiple vision, asphasia, jumping, and feigning attacks upon creatures seen by the "mad one" are similar to reports by Reay. Sexual delusions and patterned lewdness reported by Reay were not observed by Nelson among the Kaimbi. Roger Heim, the famous French mycologist, identified all of the *nonda* encountered by Reay after the team of Reay, Heim, and Wasson revisited the Wahgi for three weeks in 1963. This team found some additional *nonda*, previously unidentified at this time. In their

1965 report the team presented *Boletus nigroviolaceus, B. nigerimus, B. kumaeus, B. reayi, B. manicus, Heimiella anguiformis,* and an unidentified *Russula* (Pl. 27). All have been implicated in the manic states called *ndaadl,* which is experienced by females, and *komugl-tai,* which is the male form of the mania. Children have occasionally been known to suffer "mushroom madness" as well. Nelson asserted that the behavior, as distinct from true madness, is temporary and has socially defined limits. Heim and Wasson concurred in believing that "mushroom madness" permitted cultural psychodramas to be enacted harmlessly with the mushroom being the scapegoat. For Reay, the madness was "institutionalized deviance," or a sort of ritualistic rebellion.

Among those who have worked on the New Guinea mushroom madness, there is controversy as to whether the mushrooms actually lead to physiologically based madness, or whether it is a combination of social and psychological factors. Nelson has adduced a substantial body of information supporting the contention that it is a chemically based intoxication. Further, he notes that the Kiambi are unanimous in their judgement that at least two of these mushrooms lead to a madness that is a "bad trip," and the madness in one instance may last for as long as two months. It is sometimes necessary to overtake the affected person and physically restrain him by binding him or her with ropes and roasting the madness out very near to a fire. The delusions are sometimes expurged by dunking the victim in cold water.

The preponderance of evidence seemed to weigh against Nelson for a time, but in 1967 Roger Heim published some additional notes on new investigations of hallucinogenic fungi in the memoirs of the National Museum of Natural History in Paris. These have not been translated into English, so a synopsis of some of the information on New Guinea is in order here. Heim continues to support the contention that the temporal derangement is theatrical simulation, but notes that on a sojourn to the village of the Kondambi in Kuma country he discovered two meadow species of psychotropic *Psilocybe.* In this instance Heim mentions only *P. kumaenorum* growing in grassy meadows "somewhat hidden." This brown-black fungus that turns purple-black to gray-green at maturity is unique in being the first encounter with *Psilocybe* outside of Meso-America (except for *P. semilanceata* of Europe, which is indistinguishable from *P. wassonii,* native to the Tenango del Valle region of Mexico). Heim believes that this fungus in New Guinea is not used for intoxication due to an ignorance upon the part of the natives as to its properties.

Keeping in mind that the Wasson-Heim team spent only a few weeks in the area, we may propose that the practices of the people were not made fully known to them. Earlier, Wasson and Heim reported that the Wahgi had no agreement among them as to which mushrooms induced the madness. All of this assumes that the anthropologist and ethnobotanist going into a remote area will be given full information of an accurate nature by their informants concerning plants that they believe to be of a magical nature. I believe that such a presumption is untenable. We have had similar experiences in Mexico where searching for magic plants failed to turn up such species as *Salvia divinorum* for centuries after such inquiries were initiated. In the last several decades a number of astonishing reports have emerged. New Guinea is filled with fungi of numerous genera, many of which have yet to be identified or even collected by non-natives. Almost no information exists as to the chemical constitution of these mushrooms. It is necessary that biochemical assays be made in order to ascertain the composition of the fungi and more thorough observations over longer periods of the mushrooms employed. It seems unlikely that given the broad use of mushrooms, the presence of *Psilocybe* with its potent intoxicating psilocin and psilocybin would be ignored by native inhabitants only to be discovered by a non-native visiting the area. One is obliged to concur with the thesis of Nelson that at least a part of this often protracted madness is genuine mushroom hallucination. Even in the use of other known hallucinogens, we see a strong influence of culturally conditioned behavior that is also cultural psychodrama.

AFRICA

Members of the cult of Bwiti (Bouiti) in Gabon revere a forest shrub, *Tabernanthe iboga*, which they associate with the dwelling place of their ancestors. In the Bwiti mythology the Creator God dismembered a pigmy and buried his parts in the forest. His wife discovered that plants had risen from her husband's flesh. She was instructed by the Creator God to eat of their roots so that she might once more communicate with the spirit of her dead husband and moreover have a knowledge of the supernatural. From that time hence the Bwiti have venerated *Tabernanthe iboga* and partake of its flesh by digging the root and chewing on the root cortex (Fig. 37). Three hundred to eight hundred grams of crude root bark may be consumed by one individual in the course of a day, resulting in an altered state of consciousness often characterized by verbalization of the visions seen. This state prompts divination of illness, permits a knowledge of the "true religion," allows the fetish to enter. The initiate may be given massive doses to open his mind to the Bwiti way. It is also believed that the root is an aphrodisiac and thus cures impotency. The cults of *iboga (eboka)* use are to be found among the Oubanghi tribes of Cehari as well as the natives of Lambarene in Gabon, formerly a part of the French Congo. Vomiting and loss of motor coordination characterize the intoxication, and the attendant visions are of strong colors. Dramatic presentations of the visions include stories of seeing a great tumult, speaking to specific ancestors and relating their conversations, walking or flying the lengths of a great road, and a vision into the cave of life.

Initiates into the Bwiti cult are given forty to sixty times the normal amount of root bark ingested by cult members. This introduction results in vomiting, loss of motor coordination, and sometimes death. Deaths are taken to be a divine will intervening; the initiate was not prepared. Sick members of the cult may also be given these excessive doses in order to help them divine the source of their illness and know of its outcome. Although the French and Belgians made brief notes on a few of the uses of *iboga* as early as 1864, it was not until H. G. Pope in 1969 and J. W. Fernandez in 1972 published their accounts of this plant as a ritual hallucinogen that its significance was fully comprehended. The ritual elements of death, rebirth, the rites of oomphagos and sparagmos, the way of linking past and present through this plant bespeak strong transcultural ties with divergent areas and cults: the

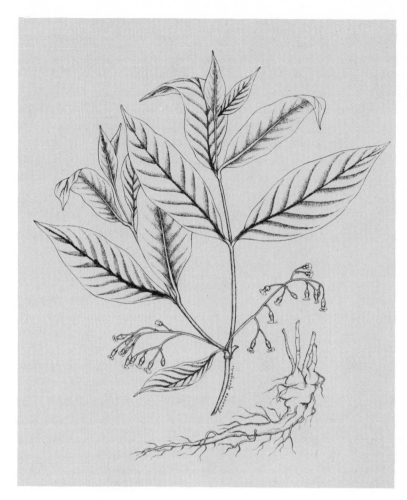

Fig. 37:
Tabernanthe iboga

Dionysian rituals, kava kava legend, peyote stories and rites, Mexican mushroom ritual, Amazonian *yagé* ceremony, and the Christian tradition. There is no compelling reason to believe that these syncretic elements were learned, but it seems that several have independent origins. The postulates of Jungian archetypes, cultural conditioning, chemical constants may all play a role, but the phenomenon is still essentially unexplained.

When the French occupied the territory of Gabon, they were impressed with the attributes of *Tabernanthe iboga* and sent the root cortex back to France, from which their chemists made a crude extract that they sold as Lambarene. Lambarene was used in western Europe at the beginning of the century to cure everything from neurasthenia to syphilis. Needless to say, its greatest popularity derived from its reputation as an aphrodisiac. It is only recently that ibogaine has been isolated as the active ingredient in the root. Six per cent of the dried root cortex contains twelve closely related indoles that may function together to produce the *iboga* intoxication. The ibogaine fraction is known to function as a cholinesterase inhibitor and stimulant as well as functioning as a hallucinogen. Admixtures to the root include as many as ten different plants: *Cannabis, Nicotiana, Alchornea,* and *Elaeophorbia* are but a few genera often added.

Elaeophorbia drupifera, which is common on coastal plains and in forest areas, has a host of names including *kankan, dolo, tulo, toro,* and others (Fig. 38). It grows into a tree up to fifty feet high bearing small greenish flowers that are displaced by a yellow-orange fleshy fruit. This fruit is often eaten by browsing antelopes, but crushed with the leaves, it serves as a fish poison. The latex of this tree is quite caustic and if rubbed into the eyes, results in permanent blindness. For centuries it has been used in Africa to cure scorpion stings, warts, ringworm, and is added to eggs as a purgative. It is the latex that is added to *iboga* root bark and may be a

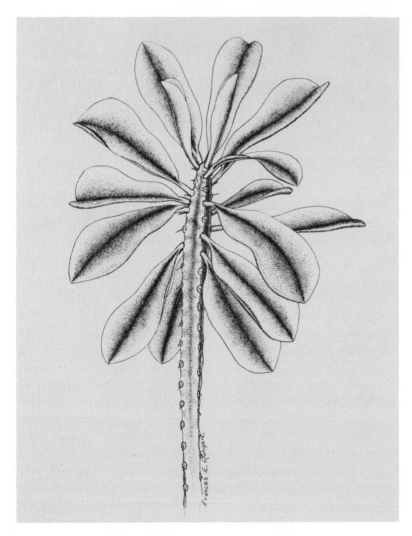

FIG. 38:
Elaeophorbia drupifera

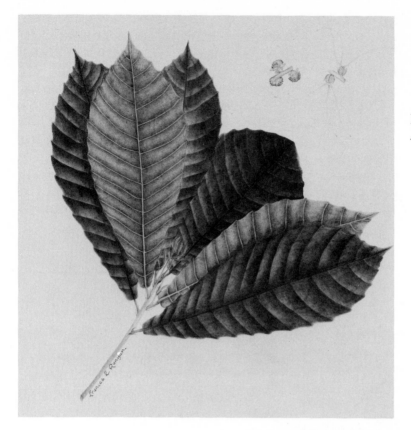

FIG. 39:
Alchornea floribunda

hallucinogenic additive known by the natives as *ayan* and *beyem*. It is said to enhance the effects of another intoxicant in the area, *Alchornea floribunda* (Fig. 39). A direct use for *kankan* is to dip a feather into a combination of the latex and an oil and brush it across the eyeballs to produce extraordinary visions. This was a common practice among the Fang people, who are the predominant users of *iboga*.

Another important adjunct to *iboga* is the plant *Alchornea floribunda*, which is called *alan* by the Bwiti and generally known as *niando* in Liberia, Nigeria, and Uganda. It is a member of the spurge family (Euphorbiaceae) to which *Elaeophorbia* also belongs. Cults living south of the Fang (Bwiti) in Gabon mix *alan* with *iboga* even though it is generally regarded as having less power than *iboga* when used alone. Unspectacular in appearance, the small tree has a root bark that is macerated to form an alleged aphrodisiac and a strong intoxicant. Powdered *niando* is sometimes mixed with salt or food and eaten before tribal activity or warfare. Steeped in palm wine or banana wine, it produces an intense excitement that eventually culminates in a deep depression known to have been fatal on several occasions.

In 1958 a report from France indicated the presence of yohimbine as well as several unidentifiable alkaloid fractions in a sample of *niando*. Yohimbine has been identified as an aphrodisiac and has hypotensive effects, while the unidentified fractions may account for the narcotic effects of the root bark. Later investigations failed to show the presence of yohimbine in the original sample, which may have been due to deterioration. *Niando* is a powerful plant capable of bringing great joy and profound sorrow. Its hallucinogenic status has been questioned; however, continued use among secret societies of the Byeri in Gabon suggest that it must have some unusual properties.

The genus *Mesembryanthemum* is a popular groundcover in the southwestern United States, but a section of the genus designated as *Sceletium* serves as a narcotic in South Africa. Kolbe reported on the use of *Sceletium* under the name of *kanna (channa)* over two hundred and fifty years ago. Two species, *S. expansum* and *S. tortuosum*, have long been in use by the Hottentots of Karroo (Figs. 40 & 41). Kolbe stated that they chewed the roots, keeping the plant in their mouths for some time and passing from an initial state of excitement in which "their animal spirits were awakened, their eyes sparkled and their faces manifested laughter and gaiety. Thousands of delightsome ideas appeared, and a pleasant jollity which enabled them to be amused by the simplest jests. By taking the substance to excess they lost consciousness and fell into a delirium." Lewin, reporting on Kolbe's observations, found it impossible to believe that these plants could produce such an effect and felt that perhaps Kolbe was confusing them with *Cannabis* or *Sclerocarya caffra*. Lewin added his further notes that both species of *Sceletium* were used on the Cape of Good Hope in the hinterlands under the name *kaugoed (gauwgoed)*, and on the

FIG. 40: *Sceletium expansum,* eighteenth-century woodcut

FIG. 41: *Sceletium tortuosum,* eighteenth-century woodcut

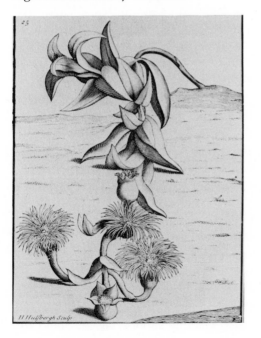

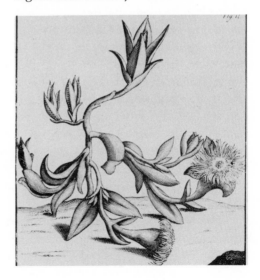

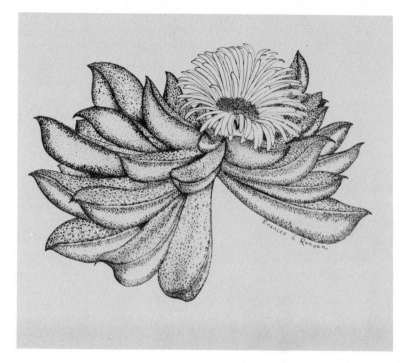

FIG. 42:
Nananthus albinotus

Karroo plateau and in Namaqualand the roots, leaves, and trunk of these are both chewed and smoked. He pointed to an unidentified alkaloid that would produce a torpor in man in the dosage of five grains. Subsequently, mesembrine and mesembrenine were isolated from these plants. The former produces a sedative-like effect. The toxic side effects from using the plants are headache, listlessness, loss of appetite, and depression. One of the reasons that we lack contemporary reports as extravagant as that of Kolbe is that the dosage was probably much greater in earlier times. Consider *Nicotiana* and *Tabernanthe;* neither of these produce significant effects in moderate doses, but massive doses have profound narcotic effects. Perhaps, on the other hand, there is some confusion between *Sceletium* and a related genus, *Nananthus. S'keng-keng* is the name by which a number of South African tribesmen, especially the old Griquas, know *Nananthus albinotus,* which they pulverize in its entirety as a hallucinogenic additive to their smoking tobacco or snuff (Fig. 42). A chemical analysis of *Nananthus albinotus* has yet to be accomplished.

The word *dagga* is familiar to many as the South African term for *Cannabis,* which enjoys a considerable popularity throughout Africa. Recently it has been ascertained that *dagga* applies equally well to several species of *Leonotis leonurus* (Pl. 28). This plant has come to many subtropical areas as an ornamental shrub under the name "lion's tail." From the leaves of this member of the mint family (Labiatae), a dark green resinous exudate is obtained and smoked with tobacco. An alternative mode of use involves pinching out the young shoots that are about to flower and smoking them as a tobacco substitute under the name *dagga-dagga*. The Hottentots are quite fond of it as a narcotic, producing a mild state of euphoria much like some *Cannabis*. It is also used for diseases such as leprosy, cardiac asthma, epilepsy, and snakebite. Farmers and kaffirs appreciate the states of evanescence that *Leonotis* can provide.

Tropical East Africa has a wealth of plants whose medicinal values are known only to the people living in that area. Occasionally a medical journal will publish a note on these, but few have found their way into medical practice in Britain or the United States. In the Piet Retief region of Eastern Transvaal there grows *Monodenium lugardae*, a member of the spurge family that is little more than a pale-green club-shaped shoot terminating in a corona of simple leaves (Fig. 43). Yet this plant is of the greatest importance to the *sangomas*, the ritual diviners of that area.

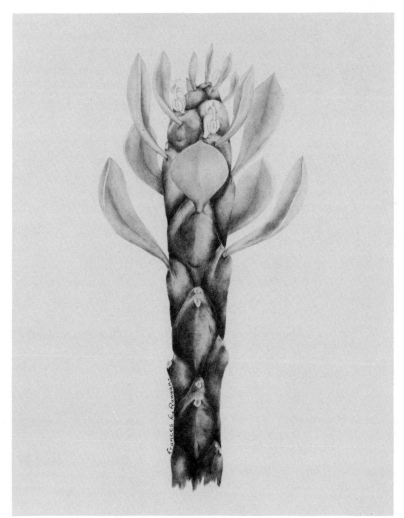

FIG. 43:
Monodenium lugardae

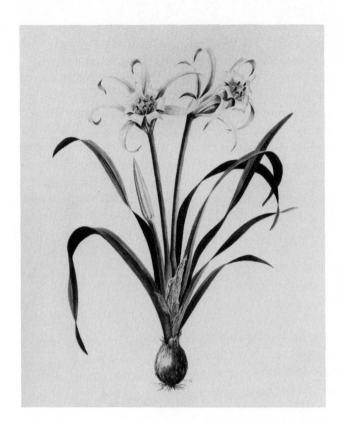

Fig. 44:
Pancratium trianthum

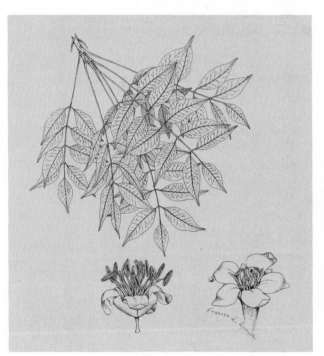

Fig. 45:
Sclerocarya caffra

These oracular figures will chew a piece of the root and swallow it to produce visions of a prophetic nature that will divine the illness and make the cure apparent. No chemical assay exists to determine the cause of the peculiar narcosis.

In horticultural practices the genus *Amaryllis* enjoys considerable popularity. Closely related to this genus, and in the same family, is *Pancratium trianthum*, often found growing around shrines and sacred areas (Fig. 44). It bears lily-like flowers of pink and white stripes on a naked scape. The bushmen of Dobe, Botswana, know this bulbous perennial as *kwashi*, a powerful sacred hallucinogen capable of producing vivid and colorful visions. The bulb is not eaten, but rather is slashed open and pressed onto self-inflicted wounds on the foreheads of participants. The intoxicating principle is transported directly into the circulatory system, creating an immediate reaction. A related species, *Pancratium speciosum*, is used by the Caribs of the West Indies under the name *ognon* or *gli* as a powerful emetic. Some species are quite narcotic and are reported to have caused death by paralysis of the central nervous system; still others are classified as cardiac poisons. *Kwashi* is perhaps one of the most unusual hallucinogens in terms of the mode of use, and one of the most dangerous. This is not a deterrent to ritual use.

The people of Zulu, Swazi, Tsonga, Sotho, and Venda refer to an attractive tree with shiny dark-green leaves as *marula* and *umganu*. This plant, *Sclerocarya caffra*, and its relative *Sclerocarya schweinfurthii*, are both used to form intoxicating beverages (Fig. 45). Lewin believes that either of these two species better qualifies for the title of *kanna* of the early Hottentots than other suggested species. *Sclerocarya caffra* rarely exceeds thirty feet in height and forms a crown in the shape of a hemisphere. It is a dioecious tree and bears red racemes of flowers on the male trees and small solitary flowers on the female. The latter form an abundance of yellow plum-like fruits at maturity and have the odor of turpentine when fully ripe. These fruits have been used to brew an exceptionally intoxicating beer. A man who has drunk of it is not allowed to bear arms. This too may be a form of social drama within a framework of anticipated behavior, for no evidence thus far has come from the oily fruit to establish it as hallucinogenic.

The distilled oils of common fennel, *Foeniculum vulgare*, were used as a medicine in Morocco at an early date to treat a variety of illnesses (Pl. 29). It was observed that therapeutic doses of the oil would sometimes induce an epileptiform fit of madness and hallucinations. This divine state of madness might be considered a revelation that would divine the nature of the illness. Its use in European witchcraft to ward off evil spirits would suggest powers beyond the ordinary have been associated with this fragrant perennial. Pliny believed that when serpents ate of it they would cast off their skins. It was said by the herbalists that this plant could restore lost vision. Fennel, dill, anise, and parsley all have similar oils, but it has been demonstrated that in vivo amination of these ring-substituted compounds can result in a series of three narcotic amphetamines. When these herbs are used as condiments, appreciable amounts of these oils are not taken into the system; oil distillates, however, could act as precursors to amphetamine formation. We know the ancient European practice of using dill tea (from *dillan*, to lull) to put infants to sleep has merit. This may be explained by the above chemical conversion.

Amphetamines have the opposite effect upon children and would cause a sedated state. These oils are undoubtedly more complex than our present analyses suggest. Longfellow said of the fennel plant:

> *Above the lower plants it towers,*
> *The fennel with its yellow flowers;*
> *And in an earlier age than ours*
> *Was gifted with the wondrous powers*
> > *Lost vision to restore.*

The host of plants that bear oils and are of the family Apiaceae are potentially psychoactive and merit further investigation.

NORTH AMERICA

In most instances plants with psychoactive properties have been used to achieve altered states of consciousness in the area to which they are indigenous; an extraordinary plant, such as *Cannabis* or *Papaver*, soon finds its way to other areas by way of early trade routes. It is far rarer for a plant to be introduced for ornamental or medical reasons and then enter into use as a psychotomimetic. This is the case with the Madagascar periwinkle *Catharanthus roseus* (formerly *Vinca rosea*) (Pl. 30). This small white, pink, or violet flowered herb is not only ornamental, but promised to become an important medicant in diabetes when it was found to contain a host of alkaloids rarely found in other plants. Soon this plant was elevated to greater prominence when it was found to contain not only reserpine, but vinblastine and vincristine. The latter two are capable of inhibiting the division of cells associated with several forms of cancer. It was noted by physicians that in this therapy one of the side effects was a state of euphoria with some hallucinations of a pleasant nature. When this information became generally known, there was an outbreak of *Catharanthus* smoking in Miami, Florida, where the plant grows as a weed. One of the alkaloids is of an ibogaine indole structure, which accounts for the hallucinogenic effects. A related species, *C. lanceus*, has been shown to contain more than five per cent yohimbine, enhancing the psychotomimetic qualities.

Unfortunately, the "high" obtained from smoking *Catharanthus* has severely debilitating side effects. Ataxia, loss of hair, skin sensations, burning sensations, and muscle deterioration follow extended use of this plant material. One of the immediate manifestations is a reduction in the white blood cell count, which makes an individual susceptible to a host of diseases. Long-term damage is yet incalculable. In the hands of psychopharmacologists, who isolate these alkaloids and use them therapeutically, they may be among the most promising of the new medicines from plant sources. Crude plant material of *Catharanthus* used by individuals for experimental euphoria can be extremely dangerous.

Datura, mentioned earlier in connection with Asiatic cultures, has had a prominent role in native medicine and coming-of-age rituals in the southwestern United States. Under the name *toloache*, derived from Aztec sources, the plant was used for almost every disease by native North Americans and for setting broken bones as well as an anesthetic in operations. Like *Cannabis* among the Scythians, it was used in rituals following the death of a tribal member. Some tribes used the plant for snakebites and tarantula bites. Among the Hopis, the root of *Datura inoxia (meteloides)* was used for divining while the Yokuts and the Luiseños used large doses to initiate a boy into manhood (Pl. 31). Known by the Mahuna Indians of Southern California as *qui-qui-sa-waal*, it was a prime medicant against the venom of the rattlesnake.

The primary attribute of this plant is that it provides the trance state for passage of a youth into manhood, to sustain a person during grief, or to simulate the death and resurrection necessary to the shaman. Only in the trance state can there be a communion between man and God. This is almost a universal phenomenon associated with shamanism. Zuni priests chew the root and put powdered root into their eyes in order to commune with the gods that will bring rain. Among the Yumans it allows a man to gain power and predict the future. These belief systems seem to have originated with the Shoshonean Indians of southern California and spread north. They are basically Uto-Aztec, but their practices can be traced through many tribes as far north as the San Joaquin Valley.

Among the Diegño and Luiseño, *Datura* was given only once in a lifetime at the age of puberty. This narcosis was achieved by drinking the powdered *Datura* root in warm water. *Toloache* would stupefy the boy for a period of one to three days, a time that they regard as holy and during which they will have a dream that is special to them, according to the account of Kroeber. Two months after this divine dream, the boys undergo the rite that is to fully separate them from childhood. Symbolically they have undergone a ritual of dying and being reborn that is the common denominator in diverse cultures where ritual use of hallucinogens is prevalent.

In the eastern United States the earliest settlers recorded in 1705 a peculiar ceremony that brought a boy to manhood through the use of *Datura stramonium*, then known as James Town Weed and later jimsonweed. The unfamiliarity of Robert Beverly with the "thorn apple" that turned a group of soldiers into "natural fools" for eleven days would seem to reinforce the belief that this species of *Datura* was of New World origin. The Algonquin tribe of the eastern woodlands used *wysocean*, *Datura stramonium* root in solution, to keep their initiates into manhood intoxicated for eighteen to twenty days. If at the end of this time they had any recall of the earlier life as a child, a second such ordeal was necessary. A stronger dose would be given if such were necessary, and this would more frequently result in the death of the initiate. In either case, so prolonged a period of trance would require that the boy be given numerous doses of the solution. Resemblances between the eastern and western rites are very strong.

A rhizomatous perennial common throughout moist temperate regions of North America and Europe is the sweet flag, *Acorus calamus* (Fig. 46). Oils found in the thick rhizome have a fragrance reminiscent of patchouli oil, and for that reason are sometimes harvested to be used in perfumes. On both continents it has had a history in medicine as a stomachic and carminative as well as being a palatable vegetable when roasted. Europeans have also been known to candy the sliced rhizome as one would ginger. Hoffer and Osmond reported on Indians who used the

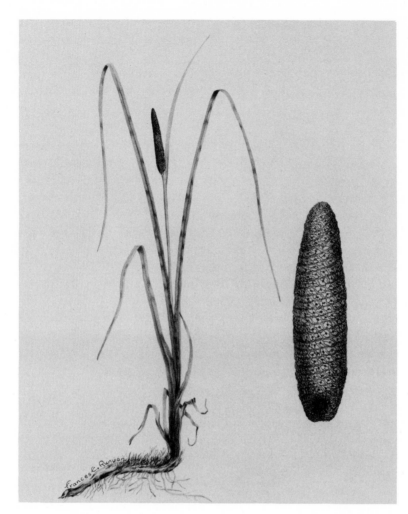

Fig. 46:
Acorus calamus

root to alleviate fatigue on long treks. Some users have described themselves as walking above the ground. Experiments with naive subjects demonstrated an LSD-like experience when they were given the oil expressed from the root. Strong visual hallucinations accompany this experience. Asarone and beta-asarone seem to be responsible for the effects. They do have a chemical structure that suggests mescaline; however, when asarone alone is administered, the psychotomimetic effects have not been demonstrated. Asarone can form tri-methoxy-amphetamine in vivo by amination. This does not happen regularly. The potency of this oil from the rhizome, measured as the quotient of the effective dose of mescaline divided by the effective dose of asarone determined by human titration is eighteen (assuming 3.75 milligrams per kilogram as a base). The Cree Indians of Canada have long used this fragrant rhizome that still eludes the chemist in his attempt to characterize the chemical combinations that create the effects of a hallucinogen.

The ethnobotany of the Hopi, so well documented by Alfred Whiting, makes mention of a divinatory root belonging to the four o'clock family (Nyctaginaceae). Growing on hillsides at elevations of 2,500 to 6,500 feet in Arizona, *Mirabilis multiflora (Quamoclidon multiflorum)* extends into Utah, Colorado, and north Mexico (Pl. 32). Among the rocks and shrubs, one encounters this spreading plant with bright magenta flowers nestled in dark green foliage. The Hopis used the root for stomach ailments, but a Hopi "medicine man" uses a large amount of *so'ksi* or *so'kya* by chewing on the root. This allows him to make his diagnosis and permits the expulsion of evil spirits in his patient. Chemical analyses are lacking to confirm this alleged intoxication.

MEXICO AND CENTRAL AMERICA

According to a myth of ancient Greece, in Hades there was a river named Lethe, whose waters when drunk induced forgetfulness and oblivion. In the highlands of Mexico, the natives have found a Lethean draught in the foliage of an attractive shrub, *Heimia salicifolia* (Pl. 33). Although the plant has a range that extends north to Mexico and south to northern South America, it is used only in Mexico. An intoxicating beverage *sinicuichi* is prepared by crushing the wilted leaves in water and putting the juice in the sun for about three days to ferment. A cup of this beverage produces a vision that is typically overcast in yellow, and for this reason it is sometimes known by the name "plant of the yellow vision." A mild euphoria overcomes the participant and microscopia (microspia) accompanies the visionary state. Auditory hallucinations are common, and they may consist of sound displacement or the total exclusion of sounds. In this state it is believed that there is a psychic regression to earlier events, and the supernatural effects extend to recollection that goes beyond normal recall. There is apparently no hangover or any other unpleasant side effects. The rather immediate sensation of cold, hypothermia, soon passes. As *herva da vida*, the plant figures prominently in folk medicine in several areas. *Heimia myrtifolia* and *H. syphilitica* are treated as geographical variants of this species and as such probably do not deserve specific rank.

Diaz advanced the suggestion that *sinicuichi* is of Náhuatl origin as it is known also as *sinicuitl*, which may devolve from *xonocuilli* of the Aztecs. No entry under this name is to be found in the Badianus Codex, but the possibility of this being a plant of the Aztecs is certainly intriguing, for *sinicuichi (sinicuil, sinicuiche,* or *sinicuilche)* refers to other narcotic plants such as *Erythrina, Piscidia,* and *Rhynchosia.* The linguistic and ethnobotanical implications should be investigated.

Three investigators have shown the following alkaloids present in *Heimia* leaves: cryogenine (vertine), lythrine, heimine, sinine, lythridine, nesodine, and lyofoline. The most active of these would seem to be cryogenine, which is anti-cholinergic, anti-spasmodic, and tranquilizing. None of these attributes totally characterizes the hallucinogenic state induced by the fermented leaf in water. Experiments have shown additional medical attributes of stabilizing blood pressure and relieving experimentally induced anxiety states. Since the plant is a fairly common ornamental shrub in the southwestern states, its popularity as a legal hallucinogen has grown, and information on it is widely circulated.

"Peyote" is a corruption of the word *peyotl*, which in Náhuatl means silk cocoon or caterpillar's cocoon according to the 1571 *Vocabulario* of Alonso de Molina. The reference doubtless refers to the wooly center and interior of the plants *Lophophora williamsii* and *L. diffusa* (Pl. 34). The earlier species designation of *L. lewinii* as distinct from *L. williamsii* was made by Hennings of the Botanical Museum in Berlin, who treated both as being of the genus *Anhalonium*. Hennings' identification was later regarded as being in error, as he worked with a dried specimen and his identification was taken to be an age variant. Hennings himself had doubts about his ability to make a morphological distinction between the two. However, in 1898 Charles H. Thompson of the Missouri Botanical Gardens grew both species and decided that based upon living specimens, *L. lewinii* was "no more than an unusual form of *L. williamsii*. . . ." More recently, chemical characterizations support the treatment of the genus as being comprised of two variants that may be treated as species or subspecies, *L. williamsii* and *L. diffusa*. The latter, taken to be the ancestral species, may be morphologically distinguished with little difficulty. Indians of Mexico have names for four different variants they are able to distinguish in their own taxonomies. Some botanists would propose these ecotypes as four or five subspecies.

An unfortunate aspect of the use of the term peyote *(peyotl)* is that it is broadly applied in Mexico to diverse genera and species of cacti: *Strombocactus disciformis, Astrophytum asterias, Roseocactus (Ariocarpus) fissuratus,* and *Pelecyphora aselliformis.* That is not to say that all of these species are psychotomimetics, but alkaloids have been found in all but *Strombocactus*. In 1972 I reported on the efficacy of ingested *Pelecyphora aselliformis,* and subsequently it was determined that this species contained small amounts of the active alkaloid mescaline (Pl. 35). To confuse the matter even more, the composite *Cacalia cordiofolia* and the succulent *Dudleya (Cotyledon) caespitosa* are also known as peyote and have no active principles. The importance of Latin binomials is made evident in this excess verbiage created through the use of a common name. There is no doubt, however, that the sacred *peyotl* of the Aztecs was *Lophophora* and that it served as mediator between these people and their gods.

Lophophora is a singularly unimpressive plant appearing as a grey-green knob about the size of a golfball or baseball except for the large taproot, which is most of the plant. Traditional gathering practices involved removing the above-ground portion from the taproot, which would permit cloning and the subsequent emergence of many cacti where there had been only one. Contemporaneous uprooting of these plants threatens to eliminate these two species from their habitats, which would take a sacrament from people who employed this plant in a sacred context before Christianity was known in the New World. After successfully holding out against both religious and legal authority for over four hundred years, it would be a tragedy to deprive these people of a sacrament by rapacious gathering on the part of individuals who do not understand the threat that they pose to the religious and social structure of Indians of North America. Canadian/US use of peyote was not widespread until the end of the nineteenth century. Among the Tarahumara, Cora, and Huichol Indians of Mexico, the practice is ancient, deriving from the Chichimecas and Toltecs of 300 B.C.

In the mid-sixteenth century, Sahagún, author of the Florentine Codex, spoke of the Teochichimekas (genuine Chichimekas) who knew of *peyotl* and used it to see frightful visions. Their meetings at night were followed the next day by copious tears and the return of reason. Sahagún indicated that these people were given courage by the plant and that they believed that it protected them from danger, hunger, and thirst. He failed to see the religious context. Greater interpretation was given by Francisco Hernández, personal physician to the King of Spain. In his account of 1576 we read: "this root [sic] scarcely issues forth, but conceals itself in the ground as though unwilling to harm those who may discover and eat it." He believed it to be harmful to both men and women, who upon devouring it are able to foresee and predict things. This was, of course, taken to be satanic trickery and deceit that would have to be eliminated to protect the sanctity of the eucharist. It was also necessary to make inquiries about such practices in the confessional. Thus, in *The Road to Heaven* by Father Nicholas de Leon, the priest is to ask the penitent: "Do you suck the blood of others? Do you go about at night to invoke the aid of demons? Have you taken peyotl or given it to others to drink in order to discover secrets or the whereabouts of stolen or lost property?" The eating of peyote was equated with cannibalism, but the pragmatism of the Catholic Church prompted a compromise of sorts so that by the year 1692 the Coahuila Indians had established a mission under the name of *El Santo de Jesus Peyotes*, indicating that the plant was tolerated if not accepted. The plants were brought to the altar of these missions in order to further sanctify them, and the traditions became inextricably enmeshed in most areas. By 1900 Lumholtz documented the Christian elements in the peyote rites among the Huichol. This work was extended by Myerhoff and Furst, resulting in a film that preserves many of the elements that will undoubtedly be lost in a few more decades. The Huichols become the most important link in this tradition in that, as Furst has pointed out, they remained relatively autonomous from colonial military rule and ecclesiastical pressures. As a generalization, one may say that the peoples of Meso-America have preserved more of the elaborate pre-Conquest ritual than have the Indians of North America.

Ceremonies that have developed around the use of peyote are diverse, and yet they have several aspects in common. There is always a fire burning, groups rather than individuals partake of the sacred plant, chanting and singing go on continuously except for a sermon in most North American tribes which ends the ceremony. During the ritual as many as sixty-four "buttons" may be consumed, although the usual number is from four to twelve. The "buttons" are formed by slicing and drying the above-ground portions of the plant. This fibrous slice will dissolve in the mouth, except for the fibers, and is usually swallowed whole. Sometimes these are soaked in water and the liquid is consumed. Chewing the button to break it down is less common. Perhaps the most intriguing mode of use comes from a report given by Timothy Knab to Peter Furst in which Huichol shamans take an infusion of peyote rectally by the use of a deer bladder and a femur bone. Clysters have been used in diverse areas of the world for ritual intoxication involving *Datura, Nicotiana, Anadenanthera, Banisteriopsis,* and *Agave.* The reason is usually to avoid the physical discomfort of ingesting material that is basically unpleasant. Among the Algonquins the protracted *Datura* intoxication was more easily achieved by maintaining the state through enemas. It would be very difficult to get a person in a trance state to drink without aspiration or other problems, whereas the clyster presents a simple solution. Occasionally fresh peyote juice is consumed when the plant is encountered in the field. Dried or fresh, it is always bitter and astringent, and the initiate is likely to suffer nausea, anorexia, and insomnia as well as feeling a dull headache. Some of these reactions are undoubtedly based upon anxiety.

Culturally conditioned expectations constitute a primary element in the peyote experience. Heinrich Klüver has investigated the syndrome of effects and found that there are certain constants in peyote intoxication that would help to explain behavioral responses that are similar and the convergent themes in interpretations of the experience in unrelated cultures. Klüver's three basic levels are form constants, size and shape constants, and the level of change in spatio-temporal relationships. Regardless of the elaborate detailing of the experience in more personal terms, these themes are reiterated. Mescaline, the primary hallucinogen, is capable of mimicking these constants and the entire experience. Klüver's detailed studies are remarkable in that peyote intoxication is one of the most complex of the psychotomimetic experiences in terms of the range of hallucinations, which include the vivid color alterations, auditory changes, taste and olfactory sensations, macroscopia and microscopia, levitation, tactile hallucinations, time-space altera- tions, and the experience of "selflessness" or depersonalization. Both Klüver and LaBarre have stressed that the mescaline experience is not the peyote experience.

The Indian participant in the peyote ceremony is shown the Way, the road to the good life, and he enjoys a oneness with his fellow man and with nature. As Lewin reported, he is transported to a new world of sensibility and intelligence. The peyote experience is essentially religious as it is practiced by Indians. Contrary to this we have the hedonistic experience of the European or non-Native American. The account of Havelock Ellis is exemplary: "visions became distinct and green stones, ever changing . . . the air around me seemed flushed with vague perfumes, producing with the visions a delicious effect . . . a kind of removal from earthly cares and the appearance of a purely internal life which excites astonishment." Here we have documentation of an experience that is not considerably different from some of the accounts of hashish eaters and similar also to mushroom intoxication.

Thus, despite constants, the experience is dictated in great part by what the individual brings to it. For the Indians it is a very sacred experience. Contrary to the ethnocentric assertion of Lewin that it "brings the Indian out of his apathy and unconsciously lead[s] him to superior spheres of perception, and he is subjected to the same impressions as the cultivated European . . .," we may say that the understanding of their environment by Native Americans surpasses that of the non-native who seeks to modify it rather than attain a more profound understand- ing. It is precisely this lack of perception by the non-native that led a group of North American Indians to petition the Supreme Court of the United States in order to preserve their sacrament. This culminated in the founding of the Native Church of North America in which peyote remains as the central sacrament to promote this contemplative state of introspection and union with God, man, and nature. It permits a return to the principles of a people who have been rightfully disenchanted by a way of life that has been forced upon them by non-natives. No elaborate tests or measurements will reveal the impact that peyote has in these age-old rituals. Even when used as a medicine, it cannot be understood only as a therapeutic agent; peyote remains sacred as a source of life and power. Other mescaline-containing cacti used ritualistically may be found in the section on South America.

Mescaline is a name that was given to the most active alkaloid isolated from *Lophophora* by Heffter in 1894. The choice was perhaps unfortunate in that it derives from the Náhuatl *mexcalli* indicating the *Agave americana* (also called century plant or maguey). From this Aztec word there arose the Mexican term *mezcal* (mescal), designating alcoholic beverages made from several species of *Agave*. Also at a very early date, the practice of putting the red bean-like seeds of *Sophora secundiflora* in *mezcal* to make it more intoxicating was a common practice (Pl. 36). These seeds from the shrubby legume *Sophora* became known as mescal and *mezcal* because of their use as a narcotic adulterant of the alcoholic beverage derived from the *Agave*. The term mescal was adopted by Heffter, because it was in early use to characterize dried slices of peyote, which were "mescal buttons," just as the *Sophora* seeds were "mescal beans." It would seem that the practice of wearing mescal seeds sewn on a peyote leader's vestments would explain the etymological connection. Peyote gradually replaced the mescal bean as the hallucinogen of preference among the people of north Mexico and the United States, because it is less toxic than *Sophora* seeds, which contain cystine. Cystine is a toxic pyrridine that is closely related to nicotine and is found in several other legumes that are used for ritual intoxication. It produces nausea, convulsions, and some-times death. Evidence for the association between the peyote ritual and the *Sophora* ceremonies may be found on the garments of the peyote leader among the Kiowa Indians. Some of the Plains Indians still consume the bean, but the practice is diminishing. One half of a bean is enough to intoxicate.

Archaeological sites dating before A.D. 1000 suggest a ceremonial use of *Sophora* seed or mescal beans. Among the Plains Indians mescal beans have been used as a divinatory agent to predict, as a vision-inducing agent in initiation rites, and as a stimulant and ritual emetic in other ceremonies. As early as 1539, the Spanish explorer Cabeza de Vaca mentions mescal beans as an article of barter among the Texas Indians, and in 1820 the Stephen Long expedition reported that the Arapaho and Iowa Indians were using the beans as a medicine and a narcotic. Both the Kikapooh and Comanche tribes used an infusion of *Sophora* seed for earache and eye diseases. These magical beans are said to have sexes and to breed. If one puts aside a dozen beans, he should not be surprised to return to this same cache and find several dozen beans. Being magical, they were treated as amulets and when worn, they protected the wearer against bodily harm.

In the spring the Iowas roasted the beans by a fire until the coral orange color turned to yellow. Then the beans were pounded into a yellow meal, and water was added to it. The Iowa red bean ceremony involved a spring purification ritual in which all tribesmen drank this infusion and then vomited copiously. This was a form of *limpia* or ritual cleansing that may be found throughout the Americas. It is more than ridding the body of toxins, it is a symbolic and physical purification brought about by a sacred agent.

Frijolitos, or *Sophora* seeds, have often been confused with the seed of *Erythrina flabelliformis* and related species in this genus (Pl. 37). Although the trees are quite distinct, the seeds bear a superficial resemblance to each other. In Mexican markets both seeds may be found for sale, the former as *frijolitos* and the latter as *colorines*. While *Erythrina* occurs in the tropics and subtropics of both the Old and New worlds, not all species contain indole or isoquinoline derivatives that present a potential for hallucination. The tetracyclic ring known as erythran is common to those that are psychoactive, and the effect seems to be predominantly that which is elicited by curare toxins that are used as tropical arrow poisons.

Were it not for the absence of black, this seed might be confused with yet another member of the pea family, *Rynchosia*. Two species of this genus are in common employ on the slopes of Popocatepetl, *R. pyramidalis (R. phaseolides)* and *R. longiraceomosa* (Fig. 47). There is considerable antiquity in the practice of using this seed as a narcotic, for it figures prominently in some Aztec paintings together with hallucinogenic mushrooms. In the Tepantitia fresco (c. A.D. 300–400), *Rynchosia* seed may be seen falling from the hand of the rain god, Tlaloc. The name by which this seed is best known, *piule*, is also used to indicate all of the hallucinogenic morning glory seeds (*Ipomoea* spp.). The narcotic in these red and black beans is as yet unidentified, but physiological testing has shown the effects to be like those of curare, further linking this seed to *Erythrina*.

Spaniards have never been fanciers of mushrooms, so it is easy to understand their disgust when, as Christian conquerors, they found the Aztecs using mushrooms as a sacrament under the name *teonanacatl* or "God's flesh." Sahagún, being a sixteenth-century Spanish friar, and the king's physician Hernández gave written accounts of loathsome mushroom rituals that "provoke lust . . . cause not death, but madness . . . and bring before the eyes wars and the likeness of demons." Sahagún included in his denunciation some drawings of these pernicious fungi and the devil inspiring them. Needless to say, *teonanacatl* was banned by the church as contributing to pagan behavior and idolatry. It was particularly irksome to the conquerors that these mushrooms should be used in a sort of communion ritual. On state occasions, such as the coronation of Montezuma in 1502, hallucinogenic mushrooms were incorporated into the feast.

The practice of venerating mushrooms dates back to around 100 B.C. and is based in part upon the discovery of nine miniature mushroom stones found in a late pre-Classic to early Classic site near Guatemala City. Progressive finds ranging from Vera Cruz in the north to El Salvador and Honduras in the south have indicated an extensive mushroom cult in very early civilizations. Nineteenth-century stones were interpreted as vestiges of phallic worship. This concept was not discarded until the end of the nineteenth century, when more finds established the nature of the idols as mushrooms. Frequently these were associated with a young woman leaning over a *metate* and grinding mushrooms, or there was an association with the toad *(Bufo marinus)*, whose skin contains the narcotic bufotenine (Fig. 48).

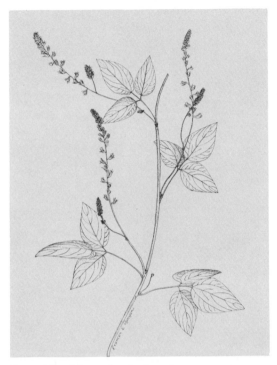

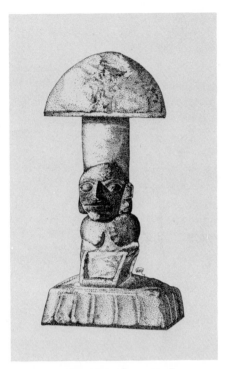

FIG. 47: *Rhynchosia longiraceomosa*

FIG. 48: Guatemalan mushroom stone and girl with a metate

It was not until 1936 that a non-Indian, Roberto J. Weitlaner, witnessed the holy rites involving *teonanacatl*. During the years 1938–39 Richard Schultes, then beginning his career as an ethnobotanist, was doing field work in the area of Oaxaca and sent specimens of the sacred mushrooms back to Harvard. Many years later they were to be identified as *Psilocybe caerulescens* var. *mazatecorum*, *Panaeolus companulatus* var. *sphinctrinus* and *Stropharia (Psilocybe) cubensis* (Pl. 38).

During several successive trips beginning in 1953, R. Gordon Wasson explored the area of Oaxaca and environs searching for fragments of this intriguing and incomplete puzzle. As he was a devoted amateur schooled in mycology, Wasson enlisted the aid of Roger Heim, the world-famous expert on fungi from Paris, and the chemist-naturalist Albert Hofmann of Sandoz Laboratories in Basel, Switzerland. Wasson wrote several important articles on their experiences as participants in mushroom ceremonies among the Mazatecs and recorded these on tape and film. In addition to enlarging the number of known species used, they described frescos depicting mushroom worship going back to A.D. 300 and mushroom stones from Guatemala dating to perhaps 1000 B.C. Their fungal finds included: *Conocybe siliginoides* from dead tree trunks, *Psilocybe mexicana* from wet meadows and pasturelands, *Psilocybe aztecorum* growing in moist fields, *Psilocybe zapotecorum*, known as "crown of thorns" and indigenous in marshlands, *Psilocybe caerulescens* var. *mazatecorum* which grows on refuse, *Psilocybe caerulescens* var. *nigripes*

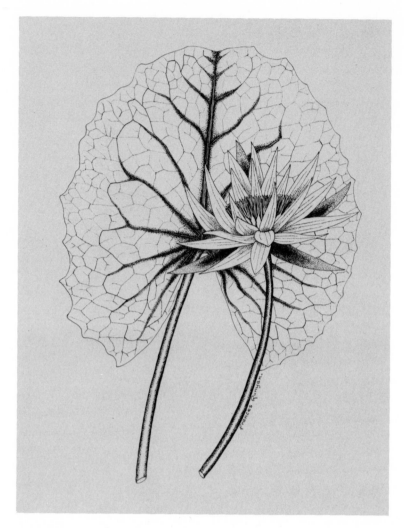

Fɪɢ. 49:
Nymphaea ampla

called the "mushroom of superior reason," and *Stropharia (Psilocybe) cubensis*, which is often found on decaying plant material.

While mushrooms were doubtless consumed in rituals over much of Mexico and Central America in ancient times, the only tribe definitely known to have used *teonanacatl* is the Chichimecas. In Oaxaca today, six tribes consume sacred mushrooms: Mazatecs, Chinantecs, Chatinos, Zapotecs, Mixtecs, and Mijes. Other tribes using the sacred mushrooms are the Nahoas of Mexico, the Tarascans of Michoacan, and the Otomis of Puebla. More recently it has been suggested that the use of the mushrooms in a ritual fashion by the Chol and Lacandón Maya may be a vestige of an earlier Mayan ritual that may have disappeared for a time and then been readopted. Although most authorities on Mayan civilizations have in the past spoken only of tobacco as an intoxicant, recent studies by Robertson in 1972 have documented the use of mushrooms by Lacandón priests within the seclusion of small temples at Yaxchilán. This, combined with evidence presented by Dobkin de Rios in 1972 and 1974 on hallucinogenic water lilies *(Nymphaea ampla)* and narcotic toad skins, suggests that the structure of Mayan civilization may require new interpretations (Fig. 49). Peter Furst in 1972 did much to put the role of mushrooms and the toad into an Aztec cosmology, and in the subsequent two ensuing years this anthropologist identified a number of mushroom effigies in ceramic pieces of tombs of west Mexico some two thousand years ago. The burgeoning reports in recent times suggest that much of the history of the peoples of ancient middle America will have to be rewritten in light of the prevalence of psychoactive plant and animal material that was previously unknown in the psychohistory of these civilizations.

The Sandoz Laboratories of Switzerland were successful in 1958 in isolating psilocybin and psilocin from *Psilocybe mexicana,* and subsequently these were found to be the active principles of the various genera comprising "magic mushrooms." Psilocin is 1.4 times as potent as psilocybin. Hofmann and his colleagues found qualitative similarities between the effects of these mushrooms and LSD or mescaline reactions. They believe that psilocybin and LSD create similar psychic manifestations by acting on some common mechanism. It is to be noted that the amount of psilocybin and psilocin in *Psilocybe cubensis* is considerably higher than in other species. Hofmann's reported vivid hallucinations with thirty-two specimens of dried *Psilocybe mexicana* are easily achieved by using three or four dried *P. cubensis* specimens. The period of intoxication is approximately four hours.

Effects of psilocybin and psilocin include colored hallucinations, muscular relaxation, occasional hilarity, inability to concentrate one's attention, alteration of time and space perception, and a feeling of isolation from one's environment. The sensation of a new reality has passed, the body is in a state of physical and mental lassitude. Some investigators report depression upon leaving the intoxicated state. I believe that this relates directly to the quality of the experience, for the new vistas, levitation, and personal revelation can be exhilerating even in a state of physical exhaustion. The experience varies from one time to another in the same individual, and most certainly from person to person. As with LSD, these mushrooms should be useful in experimental psychiatry. They are pleasant to consume and produce no offensive toxic reactions such as vomiting or vertigo. The intoxication is not a stupor, but a period of a new consciousness and a new reality. These are sensations that have been experienced in sacred ceremonies that have been conducted in Mexico and Central America for centuries or perhaps even millennia.

Present-day ritual among Mazatec curanderos involves the incorporation of a great deal of ritual from the Catholic Church, which tried without success to eliminate the detested fungi. Chanting to the saints of the church and the incorporation of litanies are undoubtedly post-Christian elements in Mazatec ritual. It is difficult to separate out those ritual and musical elements that are authentic. The beating of arms against the rib cage and thighs as well as the clapping of hands during the ceremony establish a music over which chanting and singing are heard. During the trance the mushroom speaks through the curandera and she, appropriately, speaks in the several voices of the persons she has become. A parish priest in 1629 recorded a list of the word formulas employed by the Aztecs in a mushroom invocation. This record reveals nine personages for the individual conducting the ceremony, a style now paralleled in the Mazatec curandera's mushroom ceremony.

Oaxaca has, perhaps, more knowledge of mind-altering plants per square mile than any other region of the world, and yet the Indians of Oaxaca have uses for local plant species that may not extend beyond a given tribe even though the plant may be ubiquitous. Such is the case with two bizarre puff-balls *Lycoperdon marginatum* and *L. mixtecorum* (Figs. 50 and 51). More than one hundred species of this genus may be found in the temperate forests at high altitudes. The Mixtecs, living at an altitude of about two thousand meters and above, collect the two aforementioned species, which upon ingestion create a semi-somnolent state in which voices and echos are heard. Mixtecs believe that if they listen to the voices they may expect answers to the questions posed. These puff-balls differ from the magic mushrooms in that the hallucinations may be purely auditory and without visual content. *Lycoperdon mixtecorum*, known as *gi-i-wa* (fungus of the first quality), is the preferred of these two fungi. *Lycoperdon marginatum*, or *gi-i-sa-wa* (mushroom of the second order), has a decided odor of fecal matter. One would expect the nearby Mazatecs to utilize one or both of these as surrogates for their mushroom rituals, but they apparently do not have the regard for *Lycoperdon* exhibited by the Mixtecs. Other *Lycoperdon* species are used by Brujos among the Tarahumara for evil purposes. A report made early in this century by Chestnut, who worked among the Indians of Mendocino County in California, indicated that *Lycoperdon* was a plant important to the shamans of this area in working their magic. Also, we have mention made by H. W. Ravenel in 1869, "It has been mentioned by medical writers that the spores of the puffballs have narcotic properties, and it is an anaesthetic agent, acting somewhat like chloroform when inhaled." Ravenel reported that a colleague in South Carolina made several meals on *Lycoperdon* and exhibited well-marked evidences of narcosis. This was corroborated by two of his friends. In Canada *Lycoperdon pyriforme* was used to arrest sleep! A thorough assay of this intriguing genus in all geographical areas is in order. One of the most bizarre uses for a puff-ball is the burning of dried *Calvatia lilancina* (Lycoperdales) near hives and honey sources to intoxicate bees without killing them.

The Mazatecs may select an exotic naturalized plant while disregarding an indigenous plant that they know to be psychoactive. *Coleus* species all came to America from the Old World tropics. *Coleus pumila* and *C. blumei* are both native to southeast Asia and are reported to have found favor among the Mazatecs as vision-provoking plants (Pl. 39). These members of the mint family are common in most ornamental gardens throughout the world because of their highly colored and showy foliage. Among the Mazatecs, *Coleus pumila* is called *el macho*, or the male, and *C. blumei* is called *el nene*, or child, and also *el ahijado*, the godson. Psychotropic effects have not been able to be substantiated by testing, nor has any psychoactive compound been isolated from either species. We have only the reports of R. G. Wasson, which were unable to be verified by J. L. Diaz in his excursions into the Sierra Mazateca.

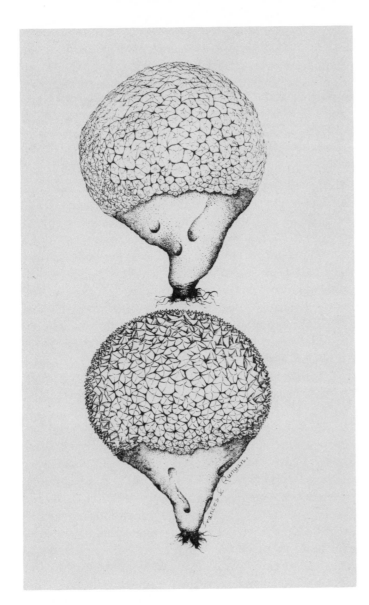

Fig. 50 & 51:
Lycoperdon mixtecorum
Lycoperdon marginatum (bottom)

The foregoing report would be more disconcerting were it not for another member of the mint family used as a divinatory among the Mazatecs for which there is no chemical substantiation. *Salvia divinorum*, or the sage of the seers, is found growing only in the forest ravines of northeastern Oaxaca (Pl. 40). The plant propagates itself by the decumbent branches falling to the ground and rooting. It seems, however, to be in cultivation and to be absent in areas where it is not under the care of man. The material sent by Wasson to Carl Epling at the University of California at Los Angeles in 1962 was improperly described as having deep-blue flowers that were slightly pubescent and a bluish calyx. Having grown this plant for over ten years, I have brought it into flower on several occasions, and it is necessary to amend the description. The plant flowers only when the branches are about seven or more feet in length, at which time it is sprawling. The leaves are an almost iridescent green, and the stems are quadrangular with wings that are crenate. It is in all aspects herbaceous. The flowers are pure white and densely tomentose. They are borne in a violet calyx tube and do not set seed even when pollinated. The entire panicle is of a violet color contrasting sharply with the white, sigmoid corollas that protrude from the tube and are up to thirty millimeters in length.

This spectacular member of the mint family is known to the Mazatecs as *hojas de la Pastora* or *hojas de la Maria Pastora* (leaves of the Shepherdess or leaves of Mary the Shepherdess). Wasson became interested in this plant when investigating an herb called by Sahagún *poyomatli* which Juan de Cárdenas wrote of as *poyomate*. This was one of the plants associated with hallucinations and magic by Beltrán in his book *Medicine and Magic*. Although the records in Colonial Mexico indicate that the divine plant was used in all of its parts (with the exception of the seed, which goes unmentioned), contemporary Mazatecs use only an infusion of the leaves that have been ground in a metate. The extremely bitter green liquid often induces vomiting, after which visual hallucinations include vivid patterns of color that seem to be in constant motion. These visions come quickly upon drinking the infusion and last only for a brief time. Curanderas have chants appropriate to the use of *Salvia divinorum*, but they have another such ceremony when this sage is used with psychotomimetic mushrooms. These two ritual incantations and ceremonies parallel each other.

As many as one hundred crushed leaves in water may be given to a sick person by a curandera, and in about fifteen minutes the ailing person will be in a trance-like state and able to recite the cause of his illness. The same plant liquid is used to disclose theft or evil doing among villagers. This practice extends beyond Mazatec territory into the contiguous Cuicatec and Chinantec areas. Plants of *Salvia divinorum* are maintained in these areas by asexual propagation. Shoots are broken from the mother plant and inserted into the rich soil along stream beds where they quickly root. When gathering the plant for ritual use, Indians avoid those plants that have been attacked by snails and various caterpillars, for these would be inappropriate for use in ceremonies associated with prayers to the Virgin Mary, who is the patroness of this plant. Sometimes the leaves are not ground in a metate, but are nibbled in pairs using the incisor teeth. The precise ritual seems yet quite vague, for the Mazatecs are reluctant to reveal such information.

If indeed the plant of the Aztecs, *pipiltzintzintli*, is *Salvia divinorum*, it represents one of the foremost ethnobotanical discoveries of this century for reason of both plant and ceremonies attendant with it having eluded anthropologists and botanists for such a long time. Although chemical investigations in several laboratories have been conducted for over a decade, the active components remain uncharacterized. Physiological testing on animals reveals the assertions regarding the psychoactive character of the leaves to be true. A mild euphoria and vertigo generally follow the initial visual phase of intoxication. Some experimenters have indicated a period of weightlessness during the first critical intoxication in which dancing colors are in evidence. The extreme bitterness of the leaves will probably preclude it from becoming a popular hallucinogen in newer drug subcultures.

Snake plant or *coaxhuitl* was the vine Aztecs used to obtain a small cache of seeds known as *ololiuqui*. Growing as a tall shrub bearing white tubular flowers in great pendant panicles, it was first described and illustrated by Hernández, who wrote of it between 1570 and 1575. A Spanish record of 1629 reported that the seed in an infusion deprives a man of his senses and is very powerful. Those who used it were said to have communion with the devil, to believe in the owl, and to suck blood. Their deity resides in these seeds with which they become intoxicated and commune with the devil, according to this account. Seeds of *coaxhuitl* were venerated and placed in ancestor figures. It is no wonder that priests worked diligently to eradicate the practice which they interpreted as communion with the devil as well as elements in diabolical magic. There is further evidence that *ololiuqui* was mixed with tobacco and venomous insects that had been burned in order to make a mixture that could be rubbed on the bodies of priests to induce what was interpreted as a satanic delirium. After several centuries of neglect, the issue was taken up and the plant was variously identified as *Datura* and other members of that family (Solanaceae).

In 1897 Urbina made the suggestion that *coaxhuitl* was *Ipomoea sidaefolia*, a plant that we would now call *Rivea corymbosa* (Fig. 52). In 1939 Reko, who had accepted this identification, united with Schultes to collect botanical specimens of a plant being used in ritual divination by a Zapotec witch doctor in northeastern Oaxaca. It was found that the plant of the Aztecs, now widely used throughout Oaxaca, was indeed *Rivea corymbosa* of the morning glory family. In 1937 Santesson had reported a narcosis in mice and frogs using seed of *Rivea corymbosa*. This was followed by some daring investigators experimenting on themselves with results that varied from reports of increased visual sensitivity and listlessness to reports of no discernible effects after the consumption of as many as 125 seeds. Hofmann in 1960 uncovered the secret of the *ololiuqui* seeds. They contained amides of lysergic acid that are characteristic of those found in the European fungus *Claviceps purpurea* as well as *Penicillium* and *Rhizopus*. Delta lysergic acid amide (ergine), d-isolysergic acid amide (isoergine), chanoclavine, lysergol, and elymoclavine were found. The establishment of *Rivea corymbosa* as both a hallucinogen and as the plant of the ancient Aztecs was ascertained.

A further study of Zapotec ethnobotany by MacDougall in 1960 revealed that yet another type of morning glory was being employed in the same way as *Rivea*. The vine *Ipomoea violacea (c.f. I. tricolor)* produces small black-pointed seeds in the confines of a papery-thin tan capsule (Pls. 41 & 42). These *badoh negro* seeds were suggested by Wasson to be the *tlitliltzin* of the Aztecs. The Zapotecs grind seeds of both *Rivea* and *Ipomoea* together in a metate, wrapping the meal in a cloth sack and soaking it in cold water. The resulting infusion provided the curandera with information about the illness of a patient, a troublemaker among her people, or the location of a lost object. This is certainly a devolment from the magico-divinatory rites of the Aztecs. The use of LSD-25 (d-lysergic acid diethylamide) as a

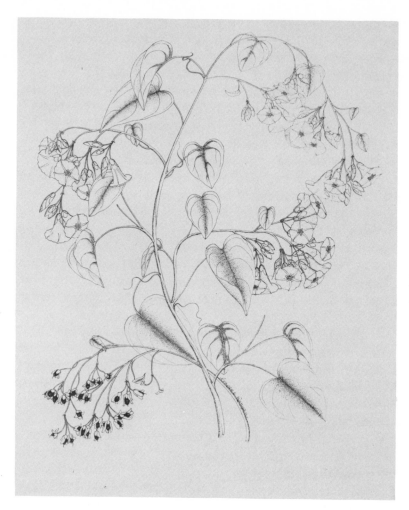

F<small>IG</small>. 52:
Rivea corymbosa

recreational drug and in therapy is in a direct lineage with these magical seeds. Characteristic visions of the "little people" are common to those who use morning glory seeds, a condition that we would refer to as microscopia and which accounts for the prevalent reports of elves, leprechauns, gnomes, hombrecitos, and all of the other tiny people that fill folk tales throughout the world. Many hallucinogens are capable of producing this effect, and one may expect one day to read a treatise on the chemical basis of numerous and diverse folk tales.

Cultigens, which are varieties of *Ipomoea violacea*, have attained a considerable popularity in continental United States because of their psychoactive properties. Among these are: Heavenly Blue, Pearly Gates, Flying Saucers, Wedding Bells, Summer Skies, and Blue Star. All contain amides of lysergic acid, and the effects are reported to be like those of a mild LSD experience. Recently, several major suppliers of these seeds have been dusting them with a noxious chemical fungicide prior to sale in order to discourage consumption by an experimental minority. Although warnings are placed on the packages, it would seem to be a slight deterrant to those who wish to use the seeds, for in a few months enormous amounts of these seeds can be produced by growing the plant in any sunny spot. Attempts to place controls on the seeds have been abortive.

Controversy continues over the use of *Argemone mexicana* among the Indians of Sonora, Sinaloa, and Baja California. In a book entitled *Magical Poisons* published in Stuttgart in 1949, V. A. Reko mentioned Chinese living in Mexico using a "chicalote opium," which was reputedly derived from capsules of a hybrid between the opium poppy and the native *Argemone mexicana* or prickly poppy (Pl. 43). This seemed so unlikely that Varro Tyler, Walter Naumann, and Frank Vincenzi undertook an extensive study in which they attempted to hybridize these two genera. No seeds were obtained in repeated attempts at hybridization, and one may assume that the Reko conjecture was mistaken with respect to an opium-producing hybrid. However, the seeds of the prickly poppy are used as a narcotic in several areas of northern Mexico, and they do contain several isoquinolines, the basic skeleton of which is common to the mescaline-containing cactus *Lophophora* and the opium poppy *Papaver somniferum*. Earlier reports of morphine being isolated from *Argemone* are to be discounted, as they have not been substantiated. Protopine, found in *Papaver somniferum*, and berberine are both alkaloids of *Argemone mexicana*. While the hybrid theory may be laid to rest, the possibilities of *Argemone* seeds being psychoactive are worthy of further consideration. The oils are still regularly used in emesis, and the ritual of *limpia*, which involves inward cleansing in itself, induces a sort of euphoria.

The uses of *Datura inoxia* and related species in Mexico closely parallel those of the Zuñi Indians of the southwestern United States, and to a lesser degree the Algonquins of northeastern America, who knew the herb as *wysocean*. These parallels have already been touched upon. A most eloquent documentation of the ritual use of *Datura* among the Yaquis was made by Carlos Castenada in *The Teachings of Don Juan*. In this controversial book we learn that it is the herb that permits man to fly from place to place like a bird. The philosophy attendant with *Datura* use is most profound and cannot be reduced to a few elementary statements. A major difference between the Yaqui traditions and those practiced by Indians of the southwestern United States is the growing of one's own herb and the elaborate preparation and the rituals that accompany its use. It may be said that the shamanic tradition is generally stronger in Mexico and Central America and reaches a high point in diversity and complexity in South America. The native manipulation of plants by hybridization in Mexico makes the task of the taxonomist trying to identify species a sort of nightmare. It is convincing testimony to the involvement of man with this potent narcotic plant.

In his *Flora of Malaysia*, Burkhiil reported that the labiate *Leonorus sibiricus*, commonly known as motherwort, was smoked in Malaya when *Cannabis indica* was not available (Fig. 53). This practice he traced to at least 1918 by way of his informant Boorsma. In 1976 Jose Diaz reported on this perennial mint under the name of *marihuanilla*. Diaz gives an account of this Siberian and Mongolian introduction finding acceptance in the state of Chiapas and surrounding areas. Three villages of Chiapas are especially involved in the use of the plant, both as a psychotropic and in a tincture to treat rheumatic fever. The popularity of *marihuanilla* will doubtless increase as the pressure from local and federal authorities in Mexico to ban the use of *Cannabis* increases. The three alkaloids extracted to date are leonurine, leonuridine, and homorunine, which are suspected to cause the psychotropic effects. A related species, *Leonorus cardica*, of Europe and Asia has long been used in medicine as a nervine and to quiet hysteria under the name of common motherwort. It would seem that the entire genus merits further botanical and chemical inquiry.

In his book on *The Medicinal Plants of Mexico*, Martinez in 1945 referred to *Tagetes lucida*, a native marigold, as "narcotic and toxic" (Pl. 44). A number of reports have come out of Huichol territory indicating that the leaves of this plant are smoked to produce a period of tranquility. Other Huichols have indicated that the plant produces visions similar to those induced by *Lophophora williamsii*. *Tagetes lucida* is also known under the names *tumutsali* or *yauhtli*. Yauhtli was a plant sacred to the Aztecs and also known under the names *yyauhtli, yyahitlm, yyahhitl*; the script in the Badianus Codex is obscure. Sahagún mentions the plant in several early contexts, and one is very shamanic in content. *Tagetes lucida* was the bright yellow flowered herb whose leaves were possessed of much oil and great fragrance. Powdered leaves were thrown in the faces of captives to be sacrificed to the fire god *Xiuhtecutli (Huehueteotl)* during the festival of *Xocothuetzi*, the tenth

FIG. 53: *Leonorus sibiricus*

FIG. 54: *Senecio hartwegii*

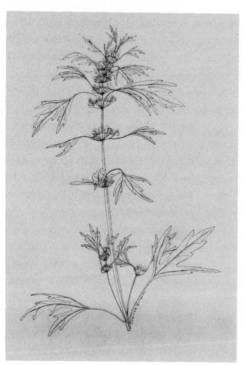

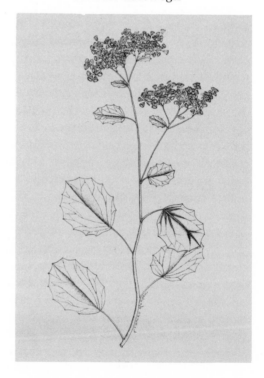

month of the Aztec calendar year. This was done presumably to deaden the senses of the victims.

Tagetes lucida has long been used in ritual purification for cleansing the air. In a religious context it is often referred to now as the herb of the Virgin Mary. The fragrance is somewhat akin to licorice and chocolate. In the court of Montezuma it was one of the additives to his ritual drink of cacao. It is difficult to affirm or deny the reports of this plant as a narcotic in that they are so highly varied and chemical analyses are incomplete. The data, however, is not significantly different from that on nutmeg in terms of the erratic mode of action conditioned by oils present. In any event, the reports are too numerous in favor of *Tagetes lucida* as a Huichol narcotic to deny the worth of continuing chemical and ethnobotanical inquiry.

In the Badianus Codex the plant figured in plate 46 is labeled *ytzcuinpahtli*, which translates as dog medicine and has been identified as *Senecio canicida*. Ramirez in his Materia Medica of Mexico refers to the plant as *itzcuimpatli* and by the Spanish name *yerba de la puebla*. His identification is also *S. canicida*. Flores in 1886 in writing of a history of medicine in Mexico referred to this very same plant and stated it to be a narcotic. In the Badianus Codex it was a principal ingredient in a medicine used to relieve pain in the chest. Vélez in 1897 concurred with the earlier judgement of Flores and conducted a series of experiments with animals in which the extract of various species of *Senecio* from Mexico were administered as senecio-toxin in the form of crystalline alkaloid put into solution. This provoked a period of excitation followed by irritability, and ultimately death ensued after a partial paralysis. He noted that in humans the use of *Senecio* caused a period of excitement followed by delirium.

Senecios were included in that broad group of plants called peyote or *peyotl*. In describing the *peyotl* of Xochimilco and of the Zacatecs, Hernandez makes it clear that the plant he is referring to is not the cactus *Lophophora*, but *Senecio*, probably *S. hartwegii* (Fig. 54). This latter species is known also as Peyote of Tepic. Most of these senecios have been found to have psychotropic chemicals of a necine structure best characterized as neurotoxin. *Senecio* is also the identification made of some of the peyotes of the Tarahumara. We now need to know the exact role of the *Senecios* in induced psychoses. The material is not suitable for human experimentation, however, since it contains several chemicals that function as liver toxins and are extremely dangerous. Recent focus has been upon using this plant to arrest certain forms of cancer. Species of *Senecio* known to have been used for some ritual or medical purpose in Mexico include: *S. grayanus*, *S. cervarifolius*, *S. praecox*, *S. tolucanus*, *S. hartwegii*, and *S. canicida*.

The use of the plant *Canavalia maritima* by sailors around the Gulf of Mexico was reported by Jose Diaz (Fig. 55). This legume is reported to be a substitute for marihuana as a recreational drug for which there appear to be no antecedent uses that can be documented. *Canavalia* seeds have been found in Oaxaca and the Yucatan dating from 300 B.C. to A.D. 900, and in Peruvian burial sites. In contemporaneous use it has been reported to be useful against the evil eye. When employed as a narcotic, it is not the seeds that are used, but the fruit or pod that is dried and then ground into a material that is suitable for smoking. As a comestible the beans are

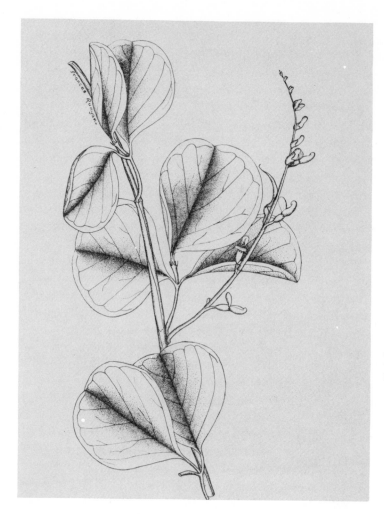

FIG. 55:
Canavalia maritima

inferior to *Phaseolus*, and given the ancient cultivation of both, it is not unreasonable to suppose that the cultivation of *Canavalia maritima* may have been for reasons of its efficacy as a psychoactive material. Analyses show the presence of l-betonicine, an alkaloid also found in the genus *Achillea* and in two genera of the mint family, *Stachys* and *Betonia*. It would seem that this alkaloid is working in tandem with others, as it has not been demonstrated that betonicine is in itself psychotropic. Its popularity as a recreational drug merits further investigation of not only the chemistry but also the possible antiquity of use. Was it a comestible or a psychotomimetic? Perhaps it served dual purposes. We know that *Canavalia ensiformis*, the jack bean, is used when immature in the West Indies where the unripe pod is consumed. The seeds of this same pod are toxic when immature and when mature may be roasted and used as a coffee substitute. *Canavalia polystachya*, used in China, India, Arabia, and Africa, is eaten in its entirety, that is, both seed and pod, when unripe. The ripe seed of this species is poisonous. We have no similar record of using the seed or fruit of either of these other two species in a manner similar to that of *C. maritima* in Mexico, and a comprehensive survey of this fascinating legume in all of its uses remains to be accomplished.

SOUTH AMERICA

Since the voyage of that remarkable ethnobotanist Richard Spruce to the Amazon and Andes during the years 1849 to 1864, ethnobotanists have journeyed to the Amazon in order to study the plants and the people. Wallace's edited notes of Spruce appeared in two volumes under the imprint of the Macmillan Company in 1908 and are essential reading for anyone who would attempt to penetrate this area in an anthropological or ethnobotanical foray. A more eloquent ethnobotanical chronicle for this vast area has yet to appear.

Most investigators since the expedition of Spruce have found a few weeks to attempt to add to the information that this famous botanist presented. One notable exception is Professor Richard Evans Schultes, Director of the Botanical Museum of Harvard University. Schultes has spent seventeen years studying in the Amazon and has lived among its people for extended periods of time during which he has presented ethnobotanists with a flood of papers that have added much to our knowledge of psychoactive plants of the area and the context of their use, and he has given us new genera and species that were formerly unknown in a ritual context. The acculturization of aboriginal peoples is taking place at an ever-increasing rate, and the destruction of indigenous vegetation in the tropics is being lost to slash-burn techniques of agriculture. The valuable phytological lore that would have otherwise been lost, and the traditions that are as perishable have been recorded by Richard Schultes and a number of his students. The legacy of the intrepid botanist Richard Spruce has been passed on to his legitimate heir.

In his *Notes of a Botanist on the Amazon and Andes*, Spruce devotes chapter twenty-five to narcotics and stimulants. What is so laudable about the approach of this gentleman from Yorkshire is that instead of viewing with horror the practices so vastly different from anything that he had previously known, he records events with fascination. His drawings of people and places are quite accomplished. It must have shocked many of his readers to find Spruce in accord with the medicine of the Amazon: "the domestic medicine of the South American Indians is chiefly hygienic, as such medicine ought to be, it being of greater daily importance to preserve health than to cure disease." He further noted that if the physicians of these people were sometimes lacking in skill, their methods were still far less dangerous than the practices of Western medicine as portrayed by Lesage and Molière. The warm sympathies of this great man opened doors to him that were closed to the judgemental Portugese missionaries, who saw the devil in every sacred act of these people.

Of all psychotropic plants in the Amazon, perhaps none is more interesting than the liana which Spruce found and described under the name *Banisteria caapi* (*Banisteriopsis caapi*) in 1853 (Pl. 45). This he included under the heading "On some remarkable Narcotics of the Amazon Valley and Orinoco" and remarked on his good fortune of not only being able to see this famous narcotic in use, but to record its botanical features. *Ayahuasca* or dead man's vine was the name given to the plant in Ecuador, *caapi* in Brazil and Venezuela, and *cadána* by the Tucáno Indians on the Vaupés. Spruce noted that the lower part of the stem of this woody vine was stripped away and beaten in a mortar with the roots of *Haemadictyon amazonicum* and water. After being sufficiently triturated, the brew was passed through a sieve into a bowl and enough water was added to it to make it potable (Fig. 56). The color at that point was brownish-green and the flavor quite bitter and disagreeable.

It was November of 1852 when Spruce found himself an honored guest at a Dabocurí, or Feast of Gifts, given in the village of Panuré in a house known as the turkey-buzzard's nest. He writes of his nocturnal arrival just as the lugubrious sound of the sacred trumpets began to boom heavily and the women, under penalty of death, scurried to hide. Some three hundred men assembled and dances commenced. Five or six times in intervals between the dances, young initiates would drink *caapi* from the gourd of the cupbearer.

> The cupbearer . . . starts at a short run from the opposite end of the house with a small calabash containing about a teacupful of caapi in each hand, muttering "Mo-mo-mo-mo-mo" as he runs, and gradually sinking down until at last his chin nearly touches his knees, when he reaches out one of his cups to the man who stands ready to receive it, and when that is drunk off, then the other cup.
>
> In two minutes or less after drinking it, its effects begin to be apparent. The Indian turns deadly pale, trembles in every limb, and horror is in his aspect. Suddenly contrary symptoms succeed; he bursts into a perspiration and seems possessed with reckless fury, seizes whatever arms are at hand, his murucu, bow and arrows, or cutlass, and rushes to the doorway, where he inflicts violent blows on the ground or the doorposts, calling out all the while, "Thus would I do to mine enemy (naming him by his name) were this he!" In about ten minutes the excitement has passed off, and the Indian grows calm, but perhaps exhausted. Were he at home in his hut, he would sleep off the remaining fumes, but now he must shake off his drowsiness by renewing the dance.

The character of Spruce was that of an abstemious man, and it was with no great pleasure that he was obliged to "dispatch" a cup of the "nauseous beverage" himself followed by a gourd full of Manihot root beer, which he took with "secret loathing." Were that not enough, he was then given a cigar two feet long and as full as his wrist, followed by a cup of palm wine. He retired to a hammock with a cup of coffee and "the strong inclination to vomit." One must admire his stamina and endurance given his naturally delicate nature, which he constantly overcame in his Amazon and Andean expedition. It is noteworthy that Spruce indicated seeing vines under cultivation at this time. Only a few years later the explorer Villavicencio, writing on the geography of Ecuador, encountered the Zaparo, Angatero, and Mazan of the

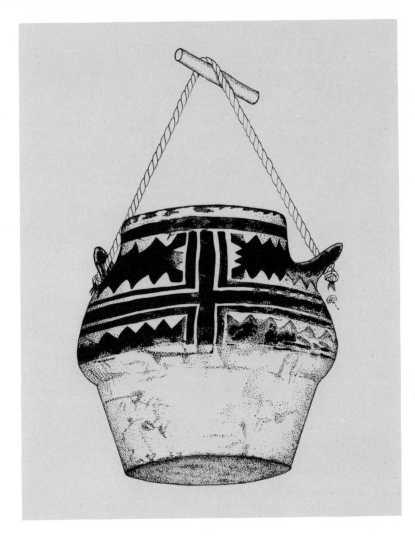

FIG. 56:
Bowl used for ayahuasca

Ecuadorian Amazon using a similar decoction in order to deliberate on matters of war and love, to learn the source of spells, to divine truth, and to see into the future. While the published report of Villavicencio predates that of Spruce, it lacks the astute observations of the latter. As a botanical explorer, Spruce made careful and useful notes as well as collecting specimens. When he later visited the Zaparo, he correctly identified the plant which to Villavicencio was only a vine of some unidentified sort. A plethora of similar vagaries appeared from subsequent explorers who could say little more than *"auyahuasca, caapi,* and *yajé* are brewed from a jungle vine."

Banisteriopsis brews are known by a variety of names according to the area's dialects as well as by the nature of the brew; many admixtures have been recorded since the first note of *Haemadictyon amazonicum* (now properly recorded as

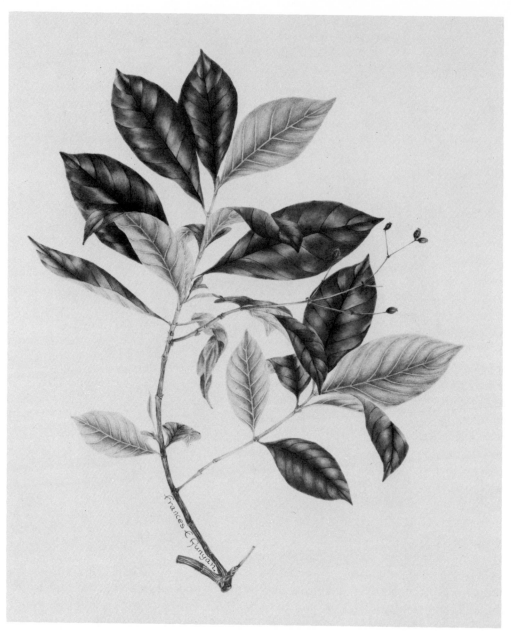

FIG. 57: *Psychotria viridis*

Prestonia amazonica). What was formerly believed to have been brewed from a single species, *B. caapi* is now known to be derived from three additional species: *B. inebrians*, *B. rusbyana*, and *B. quitensis*. *Ayahuasqueros*, or those who use this beverage, are to be found in the Amazon basin of Brazil, Bolivia, Colombia, Ecuador, and Peru, as well as in the Orinoco of Venezuela and the Pacific coast of Colombia.

In the northwest Amazon, *caapi* is used as a hallucinogenic snuff, and in Colombia and Venezuela the dried stem bark is chewed. Variously known as *ayahuasca, caapi, yajé, pinde, natéma, oco-yajé,* and *dapa,* the brew usually includes at least one of the species of *Banisteriopsis.* Most of these species grow as giant lianas vining from the forest floor into the canopy of leaves some several hundred feet above. The panicles of pink flowers with exquisitely clawed petals are rarely seen even by those who have studied the plant and its uses.

The chemistry of *ayahuasca-caapi-yajé* etc. complex is very problematic for reason of the great number of additives. The active ingredients in the bark of *Banisteriopsis* indicated the following beta-carbolines which are effective hallucinogens: harmine, harmaline, and d-tetrahydroharmine. A notable exception is *B. rusbyana* which has in addition the potent N,N-dimethyltryptamine as well as other tryptamines, bufotenin, and a beta-carboline in its leaves. Schultes has reported that the Tukanos of the Rio Vaupés have six unidentified vines as additives. The Sinoa of Colombia add *Datura suaveolens,* another potent narcotic, to their drink. The Ingano of a neighboring area add *Alternanthera lehmannii* to their brew. The Kofán and Jívaro of Colombia and Ecuador include the hallucinogenic *Brunfelsia grandiflora. Malouetia tamaquarina* is an additive utilized by the Makuna of eastern Colombia. Schultes, who has provided us with these identifications, has stated that the Tukano of the Brazilian Rio Vaupés may possibly add a species of *Gnetum* to their drink. G. T. Prance in 1970 identified *Psychotria viridis* (Fig. 57) as an important additive containing dimethyltryptamine. The previous report of *P. psychotriafolia* was in error, but more recently *P. nitida,* which also contains DMT, has become a suspected ingredient. One of the reasons for the addition of tryptamine-containing plants as additives to the harmine and harmaline of the *Banisteriopsis* is that the latter serve as monoamine oxidase inhibitors, which enhance the action of tryptamines. This accounts for some brews being extremely powerful in their action.

The hallucinogenic effects of *ayahuasca* are probably the result of the composite activity of harmine and harmaline, which inhibit monoamine oxidase, leading to an accumulation of epinephrine and norepinephrine in the individual. Many and diverse accounts of the effects of harmine have been reported, ranging from euphoria, perception disturbance, restlessness, vivid imagery, etc. when admixtures containing tryptamines are added; as is usual in most preparations, there is a potentiating effect as a result of the monoamine oxidase inhibitors acting upon the tryptamines from *Banisteriopsis rusbyana* or *Psychotria viridis.* This more potent brew accounts for the repeated reports of soul flight, visionary experiences, supernatural contact, the appearance of transpersonal symbols and archetypes, and divinatory activities. The collective consciousness of initiates in a *Banisteriopsis* ceremony has a great deal to do with the history presented in myths, symbols, and art before the initiation; that is to say, the boy is predisposed by his elders toward an enactment of a sort of psychodrama appropriate to the occasion. This by no means negates the personal subjective elements that are beyond control. Several anthropologists working in this area have provided a succession of accounts and insights that go beyond the mere characterization of the plant and its chemistry.

In addition to the above-mentioned elements, there is one more that is worthy of greater attention than it has previously been given, namely the "sexual impressions" that the brew provides, to use the expression of Lewin. The use of the drug for aphrodisiacal effects was noted by Wiffen in 1915, Reinburg in 1921, and Dobkin de Rios in 1970 and 1972. Harmaline and harmalol have produced sexual responses in rats under laboratory conditions. Five milligrams of harmine alone produce measurable sexual activity and vaginal dilation in rats. The other two isomers contribute to the effect. The aphrodisiacal effects and the sexual responses are usually ignored or are dispatched to an obscure anthropological or medical journal where they are obliquely noted. The psychoerotic effects in the *ayahuasca* ceremonies that have traditionally involved only males and extensive flagellation are worth more careful documentation and attention. Is this in part the sort of psychodrama akin to that which Reay described in New Guinea? The only significant insights to date have come from Reichel-Dolmatoff's 1971 book, *Amazon-Cosmos: The Sexual and Religious Symbolism of the Tukano Indians.* He has systematically explored the sexual content of these visionary states.

Another unusual condition of *ayahuasca* intoxication is augmentation of vision resulting in brilliant ornamentation, unusually perceptive night vision, illusion of rapid size changes in people and objects, and a pervasive overcast of blues and violets. This depends, of course, on the composition of the brew. Excessive doses result in nightmarish visions that simulate a psychosis. Curiously, the *ayahuasquero* does not lose consciousness nor does he lose motor coordination. It has been demonstrated, to the astonishment of foreigners, that an Indian may run through a forest at night under the influence of the drug and not stumble or lose his footing. The vision is remarkably clear, perhaps augmented as *ayahuasqueros* insist, and the footing sure.

It is not only pleasurable states that may result from *ayahuasca*, but certain illnesses can be healed by those ordained to accomplish such feats. Illness has many faces and, in addition to the indisposition of the body as the result of fevers, wounds, etc., there is the condition of being bewitched or hexed by a brujo or malevolent person. In either case the *ayahuasca* healer is able to divine the illness and remove the causative agent in the mind of his patient. An elaborate documentation of this ceremony of healing as well as the use of *Banisteriopsis* in witchcraft was presented by Dobkin de Rios in 1970 after her work in a village in Iquitos, Peru.

Among the Makú in the northern Brazilian Amazon, another beverage is prepared under the name *caapi*, which may represent the *caapipinima* or painted caapi of the Rio Vaupés of Brazil. Various kinds of caapi have been reported; these may represent different species of *Tetrapteris* of the family Malpighiaceae to which *Banisteriopsis* also belongs. We know that *caapi* among the Makús is the attractive *T. methystica* (Pl. 46). This plant also is a liana whose flowers appear in brilliant yellow panicles in the canopy above the forest. Each individual flower is yellow tinged with red near the center. Bark is stripped from the plant and steeped in water until it becomes quite yellow. The infusion in cold water is drunk without adding any other plants. *Caapi* produced from this genus is very similar in content to that from *Banisteriopsis*, as attested to by Schultes, who in 1948 participated in the ritual use of this drink among the Makú on the Rio Tikié and gave the specific name to this plant. It is believed that beta-carbolines, such as harmine and its isomers, are the active intoxicants.

Brunfelsia species have been admixtures to *caapi*, but have also been used to prepare a hallucinogenic drink apart from additives, according to reports from the French botanist Benoist. This solanaceous shrub was apparently used in the western Amazon for a considerable time, and is now used by the Kachinauas of the Brazilian Amazon to prepare a hallucinogenic philtre. *Brunfelsia tastevinii*, named after the missionary R. P. Tastevin, is utilized by these people under the name *keya-honé*. This preparation, they believe, allows them to fight all sorts of maladies. Juice expressed from the plant, when drunk, takes effect in about fifteen minutes and renders the participant speechless. According to Tastevin, "the magical properties" then become apparent and the victim of the drug sees visions of dragons, tigers, and the like, which seek to devour him. The action lasts for four or five hours depending upon the amount he has consumed. In its natural habitat the plant grows as a vine, probably due to the low light intensity of the forest floor, but when cultivated it forms a bush, seldom branching in excess of two meters. The tubular, greenish-yellow flowers terminate the branches in abbreviated pedicellate cymes.

Brunfelsia species are also known in the Colombian Putamayo as the shrub that intoxicates, and in Brazilian medicine *B. uniflora* is important in folk medicine to treat fevers, snakebite, rheumatism, etc. Work done in the Colombian Amazon by Plowman suggests that the plant used in this region is *B. grandiflora* (Pl. 47). Some of the earlier descriptions may be based upon the misidentification of this highly variable species that is widely distributed in forested regions throughout much of South America.

Earlier identifications of alkaloids under the names franciscaine, manacine, and brunfelsine seem to be insufficient characterizations, as does the coumarin, scopoletin. The action of the leaves and bark in an infusion suggests the presence of tropane-like alkaloids, but these remain to be determined.

Snuffs derived from a large number of plant species figure prominently in the ethnobotanical lore of much of South America. The practices of snuffing and the great diversity of appointments to these practices were very well documented by Wasson in 1965 in his fine monograph on this subject. Containers made of large snail shells are often used to carry snuff, and the snuffing tubes are usually made of hollow plant stems or the hollowed bones of certain birds' legs. The wide variety of forms of these tubes allows self-administration of a narcotic snuff or permits it to be blown into the nostrils of a friend (Fig. 58). These practices are rapidly disappearing through acculturation, and it is largely the astute observations of early explorers that have given us information on the practices. The precise identification of some of the botanical sources of these snuffs remained to be identified until relatively recently.

The shamanic context of use is well established and is manifest in some of the figuring on the snuffing apparatus as well as their forms. An intimate association with birds is characteristic of many snuffing practices. The snuffing tubes of tribes of the right bank of the Rio Guaporé terminate in various bird heads, and clay

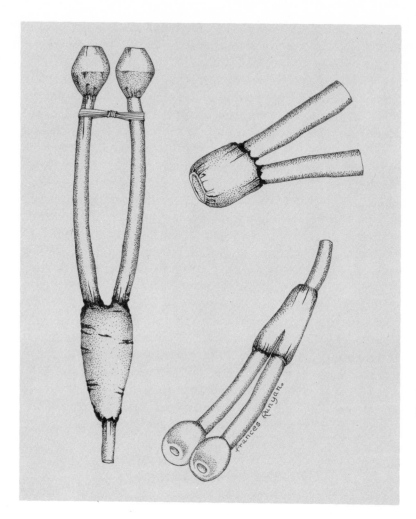

snuffing pottery from as far north as Costa Rica reveals the form of birds that is associated with soul flight. The keen sight of the eagle makes it a sacred bird in the mythology of many of these people, and the vulture, for the presumed reason of its high flight and its ability to remain seemingly suspended in air, is also sacred. I believe that we must not neglect the role of the vulture as a scavenger in eating the dead. The role of endocannibalism among some tribes and the relationship of this practice to the birds that are represented in their myths deserve more attention. This is obliquely found in the account of Goldman, who in 1963 published a résumé of the mourning practices of the Cubeo in which the vulture is the patron of ecstatic intoxication and presides over the ceremony. It is almost a dictum that in true shamanism there is invariably the bird spirit represented, whether it be the raven of the Eskimos, the gulls of the northwest United States coast, the *mut* (vulture) of the Egyptian shaman-priest, the eagle of the American Indians, the crested harpy eagle and vulture in South America, the plover in Samoa and related cultures, etc. An anthropologist might logically extend this to the dove as the Holy Ghost in Christian tradition. Spirit flight requires such a manifestation.

The most widespread snuffing practice involves the genus *Anadenanthera*, which was formerly included in the *Niopa* section of the genus *Piptadenia*, under which designation early studies are to be found (Fig. 59). The scholarly work of Siri von Reis Altschul published in 1972 clarified many formerly obscure aspects of the genus with respect to the correct botanical designation, patterns of distribution, cultural treatment, cross-cultural contexts, and phytochemistry. It stands as a model for the approach that is desperately needed for many other genera. This monograph, the culmination of seventeen years of investigation, does not lend itself to condensation. The snuffs known as *yopo, vilca,* and *cohoba* belong to *Anadenanthera peregrina* (varieties *peregrina* and *flacata*) and *Anadenanthera colubrina* (varieties *cebil* and *colubrina*). Von Altschul does a great service for the scientist by

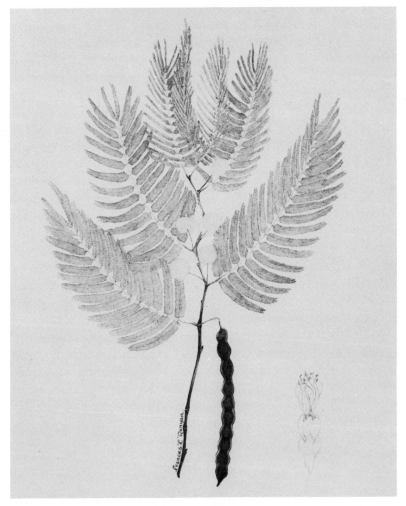

Fig. 59:
Anadenanthera peregrina

distinguishing between the botanical sources for snuffs that were often confused with several other genera and species in diverse families.

Von Humboldt and Spruce both encountered and wrote of the snuff that is derived from *Anadenanthera* (thought to be a *Mimosa* or *Acacia* by some explorers). The account of von Humboldt under the notation of *niopo* was laconic, but Richard Spruce wrote a fairly lengthy and stylish account of his experiences with the seed of this legume. While he had gathered specimens of the tree in 1850, it was not until four years later, at the cataracts of the Orinoco, that he encountered a wandering group of Guahibos encamped on the savannas of the Maypures making *niopo* snuff. Spruce watched an old man roast seeds of the tree and powder them on a platter using a wooden spatula and then neatly pour the stuff into a container made from the leg bone of a jaguar. He was intrigued by the process and purchased the apparatus for the Museum at Kew Gardens. He described a Y-shaped snuffing tube and records the reaction of the Indians as being without hunger or thirst; "One feels so good," Spruce says, recording a Guahibo, "No hunger, no thirst, no tired!" It should be noted that the informant sniffed from a box of *niopo* through this tube and then chewed the bark of *Banisteriopsis*, accounting in part for the total effects. He also recorded the use of *niopo* in a clyster, which is sometimes a violent purge. After noting that the various tribes of the upper tributaries of the Orinoco all use *niopo*, he then makes a most unusual comparison between the intoxication resulting from *niopo* and that from the fly agaric, *Amanita muscaria*. The Catauixi were observed to use *niopo* before a hunt to make them more alert and clear their vision. They also administered the snuff to their dogs!

Herndon gave an account of the use of a snuff known as *paricá* among the Mundrucús of the river Tapajoz. This he derived from a French trader by the name of Maugin. The name *paricá* is here understood to be *Anadenanthera*, but the name is more often applied to resins derived from trees of the genus *Virola*. The Mundrucús powdered the seeds taken from the long pods and made them into a paste, which was dried and then pulverized once more. Their snuffing tubes were made of two heron quills (the inescapable bird imagery), which were joined side by side to make a double tube that could be inserted into the nostrils and then into a box of the narcotic snuff. Maugin stated that after a single strong inspiration (commenting on observing an Indian male), "His eyes started from his head, his mouth contracted, his limbs trembled. It was fearful to see him. He was obliged to sit down or he would have fallen. He was drunk, but only for about five minutes; he was then gayer."

Anadenanthera snuff was first reported among the Taino Indians of Hispaniola, who used it under the name *cohoba*. An authoritative identification might seem difficult when the aboriginal people of Hispaniola are all but extinct. Fortunately, Fra. Ramon Paul, a monk traveling with Columbus, had the good sense to record ethnological curiosities such as *cohoba* sniffing. Early records characterize the intoxication as stupefying in the extreme so that the participant may lose consciousness and his arms and head hang from his body. The visions are reported to include seeing the world inverted. There is little doubt that this snuff was first used by payés, or witch doctors, for ritual divination. Spruce states that he never had the good fortune to witness a genuine payé at work. His reason was that the civil

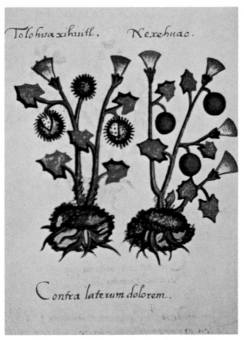

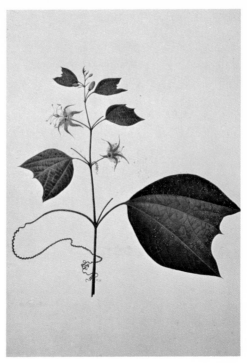

PLATE 1:
Datura species (Badianus Codex)

PLATE 2:
Passiflora jorullensis

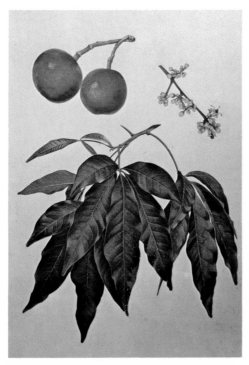

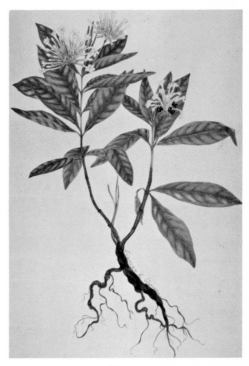

PLATE 3: *Casimiroa edulis*

PLATE 4: *Rauvolfia serpentina*

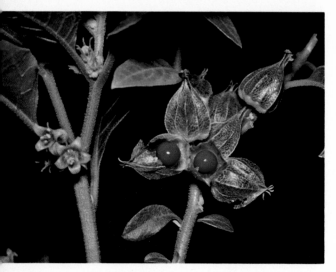

PLATE 5: *Withania somnifera*

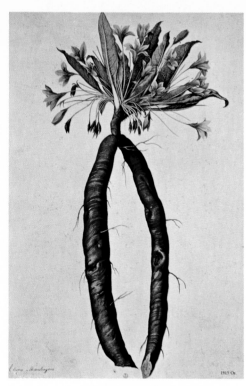

PLATE 6: *Mandragora officinarum*

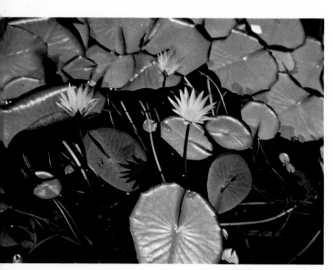

PLATE 7: *Nymphaea caerulea*

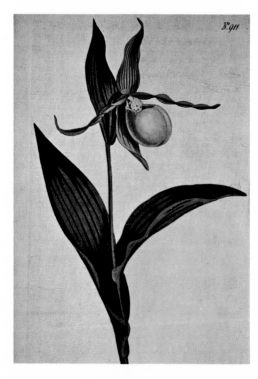

PLATE 8: *Cypridedium calceolarus*

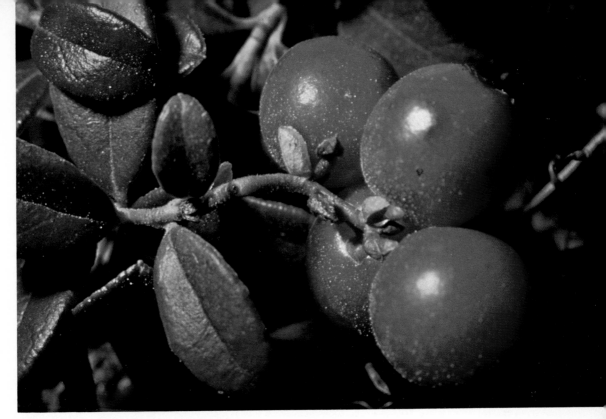

PLATE 9: *Arctostaphylos uva-ursi*

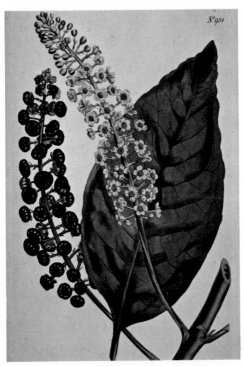

PLATE 10: *Phytolacca americana*

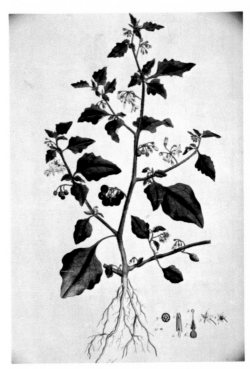

PLATE 11: *Solanum nigrum*

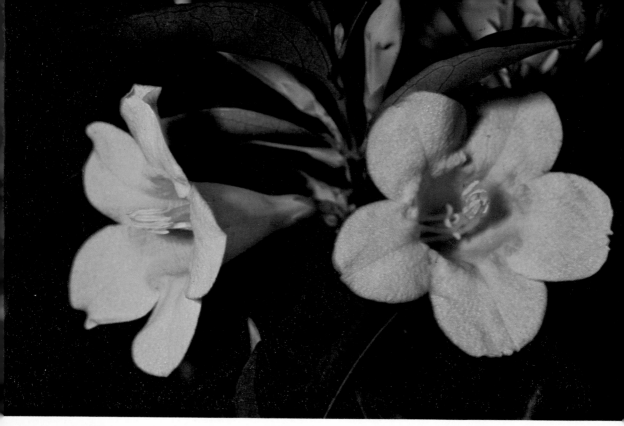

PLATE 12: *Gelsemium sempervirens*

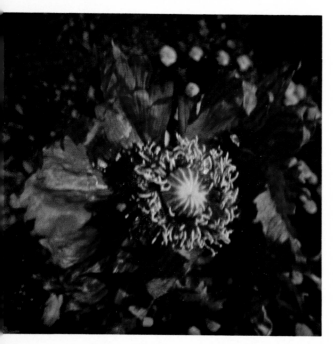

PLATE 13: *Papaver somniferum*

PLATE 14: *Genista* cf. *canariensis*

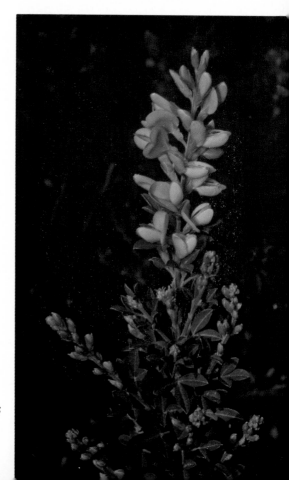

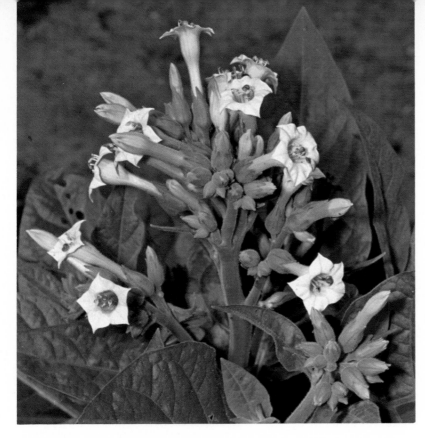

Plate 15:
Nicotiana tabacum

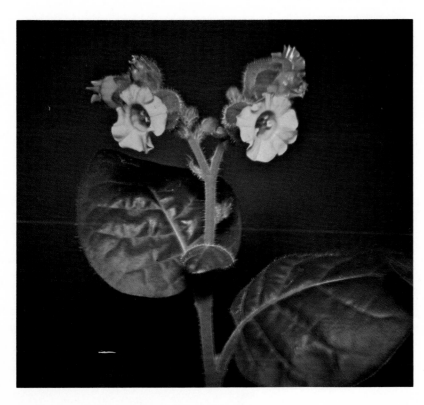

Plate 16:
Nicotiana rustica

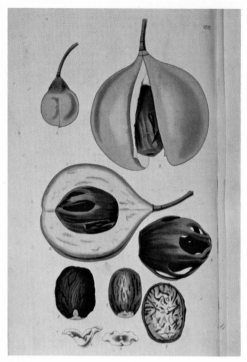

PLATE 17: *Myristica fragrans*

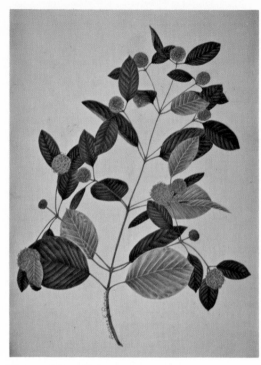

PLATE 18: *Mitragyna speciosa*

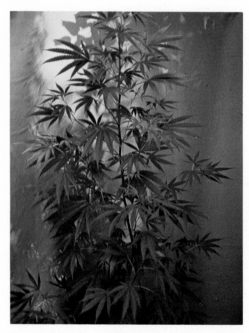

PLATE 19: *Cannabis sativa*

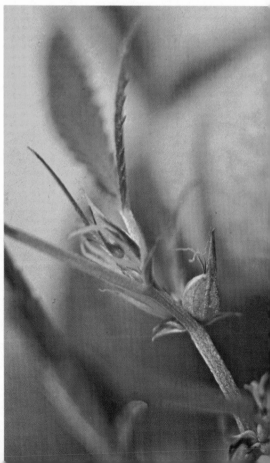

PLATE 20: *Cannabis* female flower

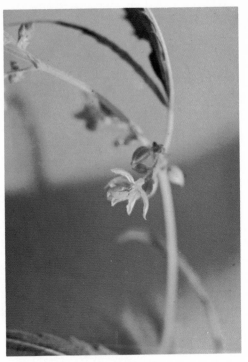

PLATE 21: *Cannabis* male

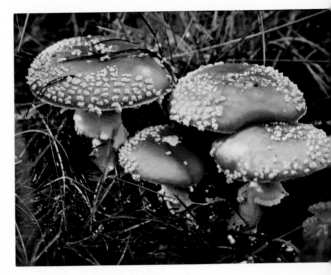

PLATE 22: *Amanita muscaria*

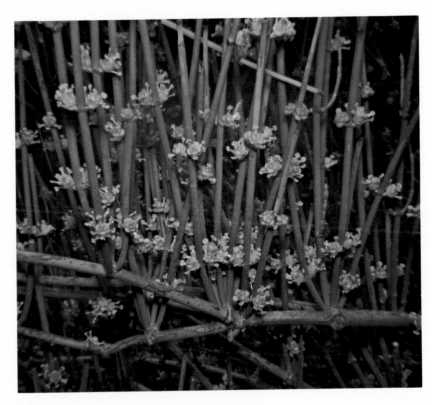

PLATE 23:
Ephedra trifurca

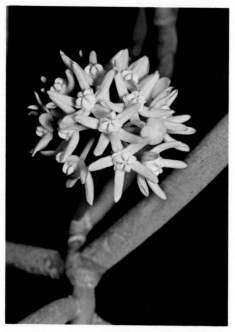

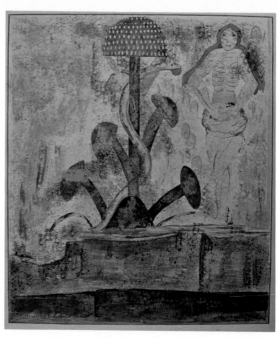

PLATE 24: *Sarcostemma brevistigma*   PLATE 25: *Amanita fresco*

PLATE 26: *Kaempferia galanga*

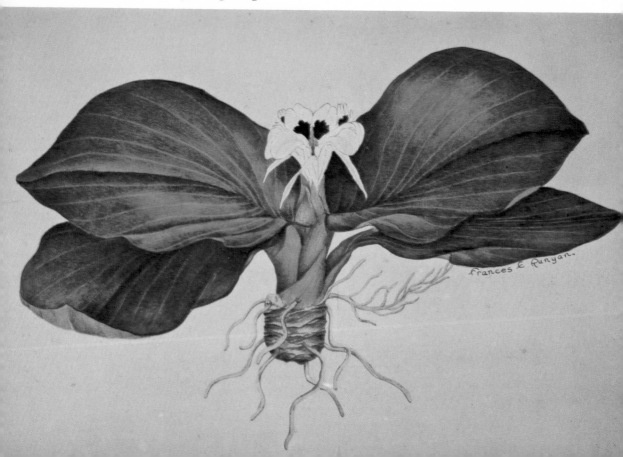

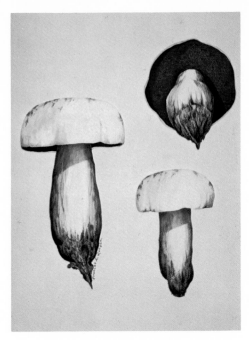

PLATE 27: *Boletus manicus*

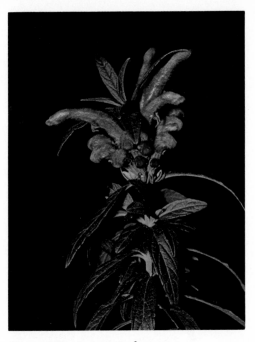

PLATE 28: *Leonotis leonurus*

PLATE 29: *Foeniculum vulgare*

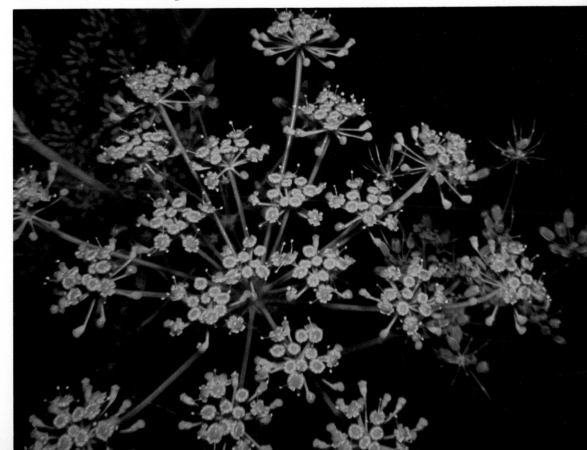

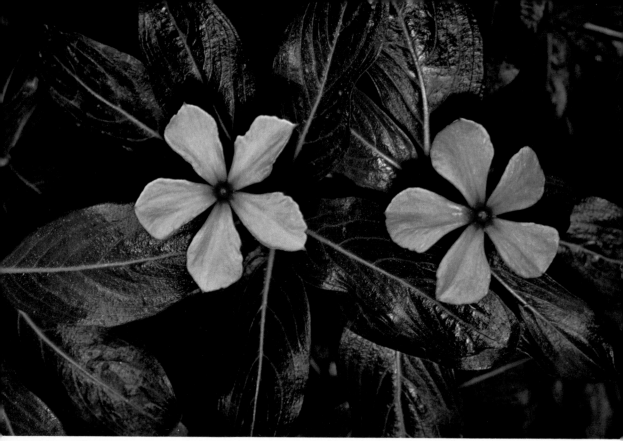

PLATE 30: *Catharanthus roseus*

PLATE 31: *Datura inoxia*

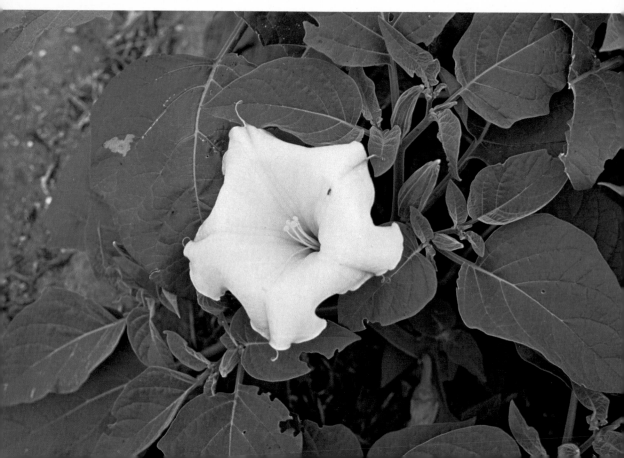

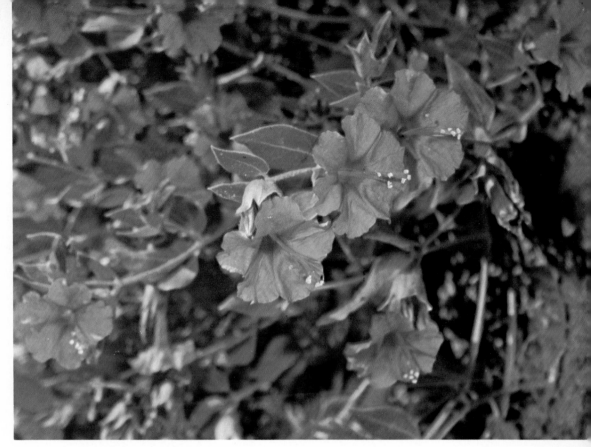

PLATE 32: *Mirabilis multiflora*

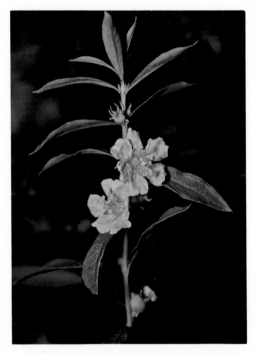

PLATE 33: *Heimia salicifolia*

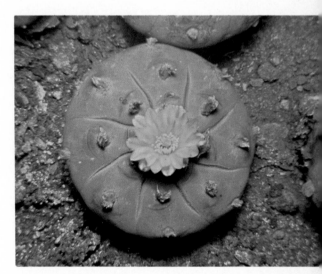

PLATE 34: *Lophophora williamsii*

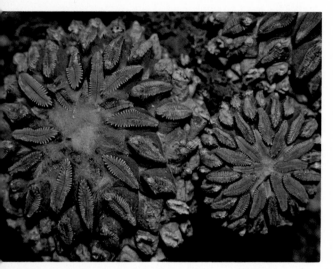

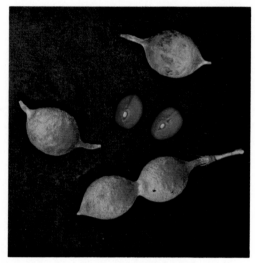

PLATE 35: *Pelecyphora aselliformis*   PLATE 36: *Sophora secundiflora*

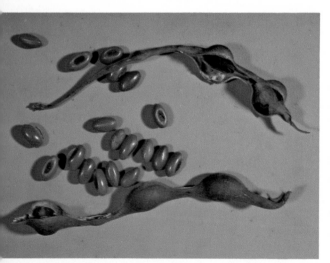

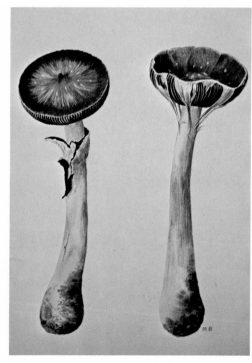

PLATE 37: *Erythrina* seed and fruit

PLATE 38: *Psilocybe cubensis*

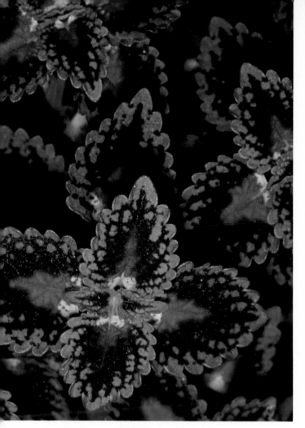

PLATE 39: *Coleus pumila*

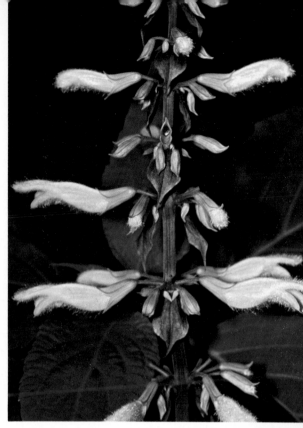

PLATE 40: *Salvia divinorum*

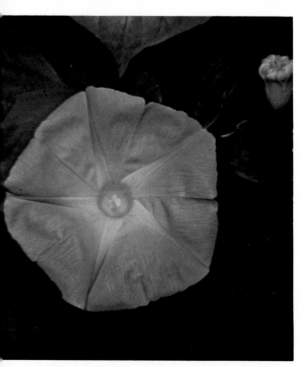

PLATE 41:
Ipomoea violacea var. Heavenly Blue

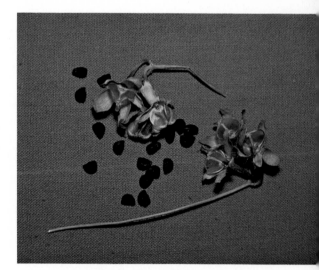

PLATE 42:
Ipomoea violacea seed and capsules

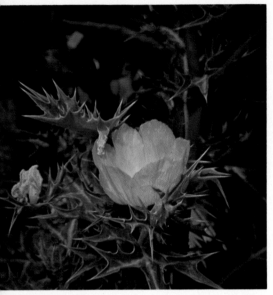
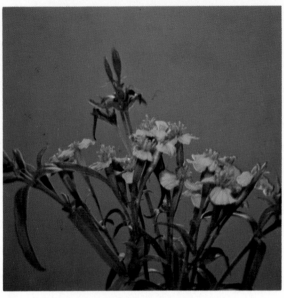

PLATE 43: *Argemone mexicana* PLATE 44: *Tagetes lucida*

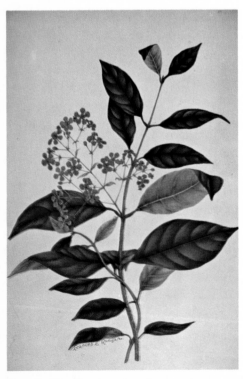
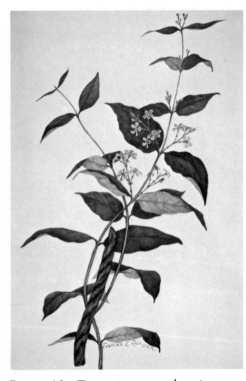

PLATE 45: *Banisteriopsis caapi* PLATE 46: *Tetrapterys methystica*

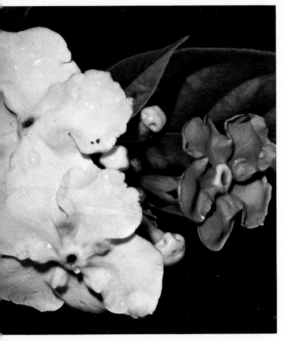

PLATE 47:
Brunfelsia grandiflora

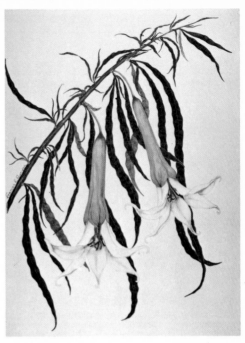

PLATE 48:
Methysticodendron amesianum

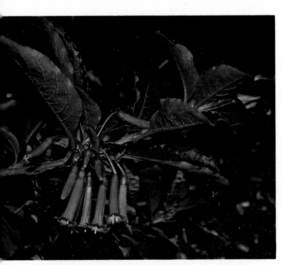

PLATE 49: *Iochroma fuchsioides*

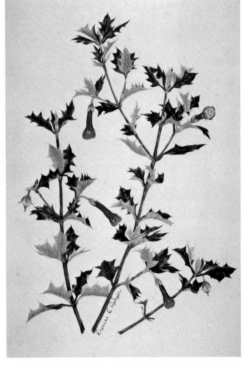

PLATE 50: *Desfontainea spinosa*

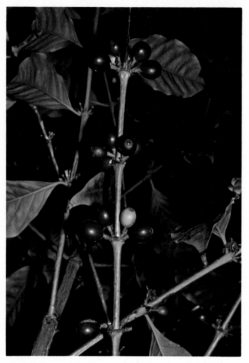

PLATE 51: *Coffea arabica*

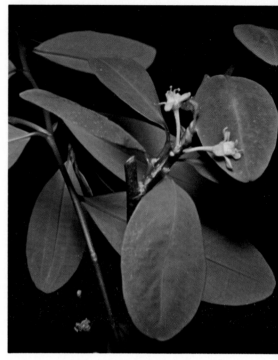

PLATE 52: *Erythroxylum coca*

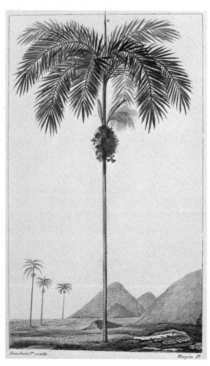

PLATE 53: *Areca catechu*

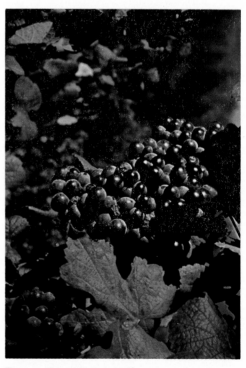

PLATE 54: *Vitis vinifera*

authorities persecuted these practitioners, and their offices had been taken over by the Christian padré. Since the ceremonies were not recorded in any detail in either the West Indies or the Amazon at an early date, we must take contemporaneous accounts as descriptions of practices that are probably much modified with respect to ritual.

Preparation and use of the snuff produced from *Anadenanthera* varies from area to area and between tribes. When von Humboldt was among the Maypure Indians of Orinoco in 1801 he observed the pods of the *Anadenanthera* (which he identified as *Acacia niopo*) to be broken open, moistened, and allowed to ferment. When these turned black and were soft, the seeds were removed and mixed with cassava meal and lime derived from snail shells. The cakes were dried and later provided a supply of snuff whenever it was desired. Von Humboldt felt that it was the lime from the snail rather than the *niopo* that produced the narcotic effect. He did not pursue the investigation. Not all groups add lime to their *niopo* preparations, and it is not necessary for the physiological action. The *vilca* and *huilca* in southern Peru and Bolivia, and *cébil* in northern Argentina are also derived from *Anadenanthera*, probably *A. colubrina*. Schultes reports on uses among the Inca observed in 1571, stating that the witch doctors prophesied by becoming intoxicated with *chica* (a beer) and an herb called *villca*, which they drank together.

All species and subspecies of *Anadenanthera* that have been investigated chemically contain a series of substituted beta-phenethylamines in their seeds including N,N-dimethyltryptamine and bufotenine (5-OH-DMT), which is closely related to serotonin. The activity of bufotenine is in dispute. Other tryptamines reported from this genus include: DMT, MMT, 5-MeO-DMT, and 5-MeO-MMT. The beta-carbolines are: 6-MeO-THC and 6-MeO-DMTHC. These chemical combinations are the same as those found in the related snuffs derived from *Virola* species. The snuffs have often been used under the same names, leading to a great deal of confusion in early literature.

Virola

The genus *Virola* is comprised of about fifty tree species found in the forests of Central and South America. Although in the same family as the nutmeg, their properties and uses are remote from those of *Myristica*. It was not until 1909 that the anthropologist Koch-Grünberg presented an account of the preparation and uses of a snuff, *hakudufha*, that was in use among the Yekwana Indians in the headwaters of the Orinoco River. Koch-Grünberg considered the snuff prepared from *Virola* to be a part of the ritual magic of the Yekwana. Unaware of the botanical source of the snuff, he referred to it merely as the bark of a certain tree which when pulverized and boiled to a sediment could provide a hard block of material that could be pulverized into a snuff. *Hakudufha* was blown into the air by the sorcerer and then snuffed by a reed into each nostril resulting in singing, screaming, and a convulsive movement of his body to and fro.

Not until the 1938 report of Ducke, a botanist, was it clear that in the upper Rio Negro *Virola cuspidata* and *Virola theiodora* were being used to make a snuff called

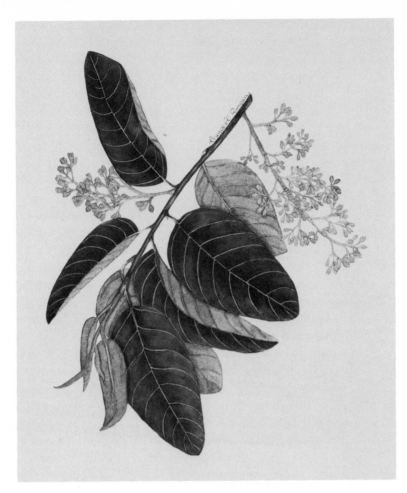

Fig. 60:
Virola calophylla

paricá. This was the same name used for snuffs prepared from *Anadenanthera*, which has led to much confusion. The greatest clarification came from Richard Schultes, who published his findings on the use of *yakee* among the Puinave and *yato* among the Kuripako in the northwest Amazon in 1954. The brown snuff of Indians in Amazonian Colombia that is used for magic, prophecy, and divination was established as *Virola calophylla, V. calophylloidea*, and possibly *V. elongata* (Fig. 60). Indians in this area of the Amazon strip the bark from the trees in early morning and scrape off the inner soft, red cortex that is filled with resinous exudates. These particles are kneaded in water, removed, and the water boiled to a viscous mass which is subsequently dried in the sun. The dried concretion is powdered and mixed with the ash taken from *Theobroma subincanum* to provide a snuff so potent that it has been known to cause deaths among the shamans of the region.

Among the numerous Indians inhabiting the headwaters of the Orinoco in Venezuela and the Brazilian Rio Negro, *Virola* snuffs are prevalent and are known as *epená, ebene,* and *nyakwana.* These people who are grouped into the Waiká (Guaiká) use *epená* hedonistically as well as ritually. It is often used by the male Waiká over the age of thirteen even though it is possibly the strongest of the snuffs from *Virola.* Any of five species in the area might provide the necessary resins, but the species most commonly found in use is *V. theiodora.* Preparations are diverse, but the most common mode of use is to scrape the inner bark and roast the shavings over a slow fire. In this manner they may be preserved for later use. When desired, the brittle scrapings will be pounded in a mortar made from the fruit coat of the Brazil nut and to this will be added bark ash from the tree *Elizabetha princeps (amá* or *amasita)* and the powdered leaves of a pungent-smelling herb, *Justicia pectoralis* variety *stenophylla* (Fig. 61). Although little is known of the effects of the *amá,* we know that this *Justicia* has been called *bolek-hena,* or "leaves of the Angel of Death" for reason of its potency as a snuff. At least three shamans have been

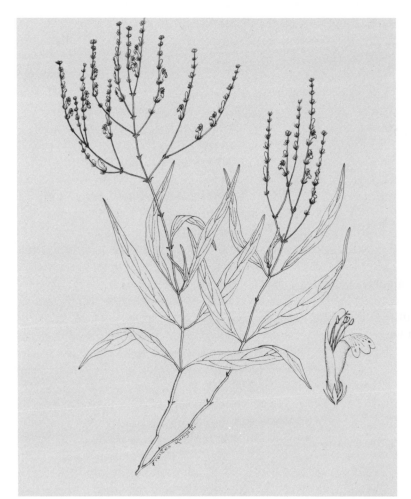

FIG. 61:
Justicia pectoralis
v. *stenophylla*

reported to have died from using this snuff from the small violet-flowered acanth. While the Waiká have declared the reason for use to be to enhance the fragrance of *epená*, they are certainly aware of the added potency that has thus far been attributed to N,N-DMT.

Ceremonial *epená* is made by stripping the bark from *Virola theiodora* and placing it near a fire, which will cause the bark to exude the translucent red resins. These are gathered and reduced over heat to a crystalline mass that is ground and used most often without an admixture. The ceremonies may involve endocannibalism as a mode of communing with the departed. The syndrome of effects is an initial period of several minutes of frenzy, subsequent numbness of the limbs and loss of motor coordination combined with twitching of muscles. Nausea may develop, but when it does, the effects of the hallucinogens are already at work. Visual hallucinations are then experienced, and among the Waiká these include macroscopia, or things seen in giant forms. This is frequent among these people, and they will often give over to vocal outbursts during the period of visions. This would seem culturally conditioned, for it is inseparable from the concepts of *hikura*, the spirit who dwells in the *Virola* tree. This is a notion common also to the Bwiti of equatorial Africa, who find spirits resident in the *Alchornea floribunda* tree. Further evidence for this as a conditioned response is the evidence from the Witotos, Bora, and the Muinane tribes in Amazonian Colombia, who use the same species as an oral hallucinogen, rolling the boiled resin with the ash of *Gustavia poeppigiana*. Three to six pellets the size of coffee beans induce a hallucinatory experience of several hours in which "little people" are seen and clarification of problems comes. The contrasting visions, one small, the other large, must be explained on the basis of either cultural conditioning or the effects due to the admixtures. *Virola* research in the future will probably be directed toward investigating the practices among certain Venezuelan Indians, in which *Virola sebifera* is reportedly smoked in ritual dances and for curing fevers. The greatest body of data to date derives from the extensive research of Richard Schultes throughout much of the Amazon in his seventeen years of study there. It was this scientist who also pointed out the practice among the Makú of Amazonian Colombia of drinking the unprepared resins of *Virola elongata*.

Seitz in 1965 reported in an appendix to Wassén's monograph of that year on his work among the Waica (Waiká) and came to the conclusion that there was no system in the snuffing ceremony and that he did not find these people to be witch doctors or medicine men. This observation, based upon two visits to the Amazon, in no way invalidates the more extensive and intensive research of Schultes, who has given us a comprehensive survey based on extended periods of living with these people.

The four tryptamines and two beta-carbolines present in *Anadenanthera* are all to be found in the various species of *Virola* distributed among the bark, roots, leaves, flowers, and shoots. The greatest concentration of DMT is consistently in the leaves of the species and ranges between ninety-three and ninety-six per cent. It is postulated that the tryptamines are the active psychotomimetic while the beta-carbolines serve as monoamine oxidase inhibitors. It is interesting to note that

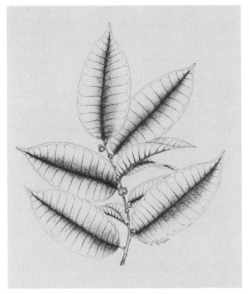

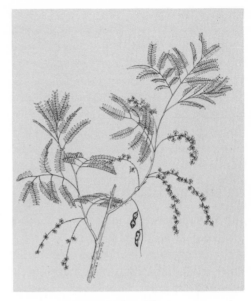

FIG. 62: *Olmedioperebea sclerophylla*   FIG. 63: *Mimosa hostilis*

DMT is not active when taken orally. This accounts for the popularity of snuffing, a practice whose origins are not only obscure, but baffling.

Several snuffs used in South America remain obscure with respect to botanical origins, preparation, and use. One that is known to have been used in the central part of the Brazilian Amazon, especially along the upper Xingú, is *Maquira sclerophylla (Olmedioperebea sclerophylla)* (Fig. 62). This giant tree belongs to the fig family and produces fruits that have presumably been made into a snuff in times past in the Pariana region, where it is known as *rapé dos indios*, a Portugese term that means Indian snuff. Schultes believes that the use of this snuff has died out, but that formerly it was employed in rituals and dances. An analysis of these fruits has yielded no information with respect to a narcotic property, and there is no information as to how the fruit might be prepared as a snuff.

Mimosa hostilis is a legume that is closely related to *Acacia* (Fig. 63). This thorny shrub is important to the jurema cult, which consisted of numerous tribes that have now been acculturated for the most part and no longer participate in the miraculous drink from this plant, which is called *ajuca* or *vinho de jurema*. In the states of Pernambuco and Paraíba, it was used by the Kariri, Tusha, Fulnio and Pankaruru. Other tribes using it were the Acroa, Guegue, Atanayé and Pimenteria. There is no doubt that it was of widespread importance in eastern Brazil, but as with other hallucinogens, its use seems to have all but disappeared and, were it not for reports from 1788 and 1843, we would know nothing of the plant or its use. The 1946 reports of Lowie indicate that this drink was prepared from the roots of the shrub and given to priests and warriors. In the ceremony involving kneeling and a reverently bowed head, the priest administered a cup of the root decoction to the young warrior while old women sang songs of the jurema ritual. After receiving the draught from the old shaman-priest who carried a feathered rattle, the youths would see a magical land filled with birds and flowers and the crashing rocks that destroy the souls of the dead: the realm where the exquisite Thunderbird propels lightning from the crest of his head and runs about producing thunder. *Jurema branca* may refer to the preparation from either *Mimosa hostilis* or *M. verrucosa*. In the utilization of the latter species the bark is stripped from the shrub known as *caatinga*. Nigerine, formerly believed to be the active ingredient of the jurema, has now been identified as N,N-dimethyltryptamine.

ANDEAN HIGHLANDS AND ADJACENT AREAS

Most important among the hallucinogenic plants of the Andean highlands is the genus *Datura* represented here by its most unusual members. All belong to the subgenus *Brugmansia* and are arborescent, bearing trumpets of white or sanguine flowers hanging in abundance among the branches. Only *D. suaveolens* grows in the warmer lowlands; the rest *(D. aurea, D. candida, D. dolichocarpa, D. vulcanicola,* and *D. sanguinea)* are indigenous to the cooler highlands. The *Daturas* of the Andes differ from their relatives in North America and Central America in both morphology and the usual modes of use. Most often, the seed is powdered or ground into a meal and put into beverages of various sorts. The result is a narcosis so violent that the participant often has to be physically restrained to protect himself from others. Eventually he will be overtaken by an extended sleep with waking fits of hallucinations and colorful visions that are understood to be communication with the spirit world and souls of the departed. The intent is to become prophetic through divination. These visions are induced by the tropane alkaloids, hyoscyamine, nor-hyoscyamine, and scopolamine. Each species varies with respect to the concentrations of these alkaloids, but they are all in abundance in most parts of the plants. Tree *Daturas* are imperfectly known to botanists because of the large number of cultigens and hybrids as well as those plants that have been deliberately changed through viral infections. The Kamsá and Ingano tribes in the southern Colombian highlands have created monstrous varieties through the perpetuation of viral infection. They have long believed that these plants are superior to any others, and the practice is copied in the Ecuadorian highlands. It would seem that most of the tree *Daturas* and their varieties, to include these bizarre atrophied forms, are the result of man's historical cultivation and selection.

It was an ancient practice among the Chibcha of Colombia to administer *Datura aurea* (possibly *D. candida, D. suaveolens,* or *D. sanguinea* as well) in a corn beer *(chicha)* to the wives and slaves of a departed husband or master, and in the state of stupor that followed, they were buried alive with the deceased (Fig. 64). Sogamoza, north of what is now Bogotá, contained the Temple of the Sun, and it was

FIG. 64: *Datura suaveolens*

116

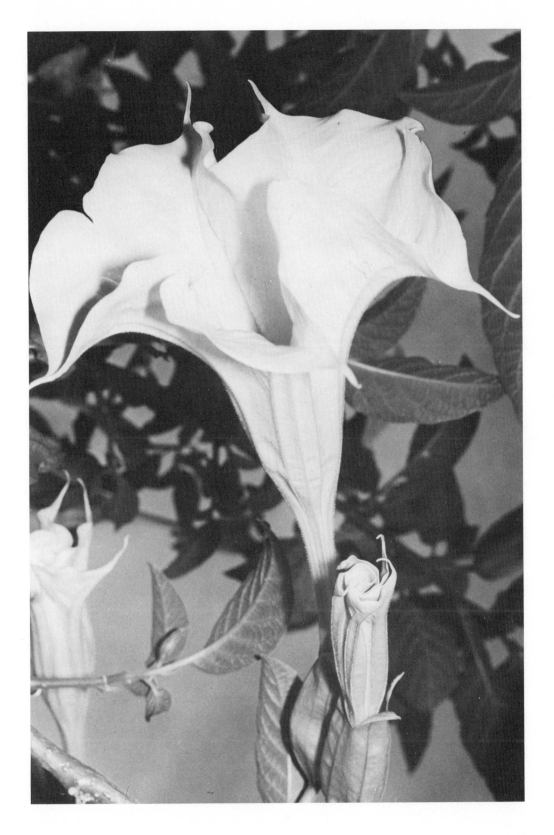

117

here that the beverage *tonga* was made to be used in ceremonial ritual. It was prepared from *D. sanguinea* and was far more potent than that prepared from the other tree *Daturas*. It is this same plant that is known as *huacacachu* or grave plant in Peru, where it is believed that the narcosis from *D. sanguinea* will reveal, in a trance state, the site of ancient graves that contain treasures.

Among Ecuadorian Jibaro, children who misbehave are given *Datura* seed preparations so that their ancestors might visit them and admonish them. An earlier practice, now extinct, was for a nursing mother to smear her paps with crushed *Datura* to cause an unwanted child to die. This practice suggests the old English use of wormwood to wean a child away from his mother or nurse.

At one time a male who was coming of age in the western Amazon was obliged to take a draught of *maikoa*, or *Datura* infusion, from each male elder in his tribe. Obviously a boy could not take any considerable amount of the brew orally, so after a time the elders inserted a hollow bone or horn into the rectum of the lad and with a pouch of *maikoa* attached, they were able to administer anal doses until a deep comatose state set in. The purpose of this ritual enema was the same as that among North American Indians. The child was to forget the things that pertained to his youth and be advised in this trance by his ancestors of things that related to the proper life-style for a man.

Much lore concerning the tree *Daturas* has been uncovered, but there is a great deal yet to be learned about contemporaneous practices and those practices that have been lost but yet remembered. If we accept this as the center of origin for this section of the genus, then its widespread contemporary distribution that parallels the habitations of man in much of South America is to be explained on the basis of selection, cultivation, and even hybridization by man to produce desirable strains.

In 1955 Richard Evans Schultes described a large tree that had the characteristics of some of the *Daturas*, but was quite extraordinary and different in many of its features. Only in the Valley of Sibundoy in the southern range of the Andes of Colombia is this bizarre production to be found. In the Kamsá language of the region it is called *mitskway borrachera*; another name for it is *culebra borrachera* (literally drunken snake, possibly a reference to the effects as well as to the twisted elongate leaves). *Methysticodendron amesianum* is thought by some to be a cultivar or aberrant form of *D. candida*, but the collective features, including the leaves, the white flower that is up to a foot-and-a-half in length, and the gigas form argue against this (Pl. 48). The characterization by Schultes in 1955 still seems to be more taxonomically acceptable than other theses that suggest viral infections of a *Datura*, the pleiotropic effect of a single gene, or the cultivar hypothesis. The tree is clearly a departure from the genus *Datura* deserving of the generic disposition given by Schultes. The natives who propagate the plant asexually (the most common mode of propagation with most tree *Daturas*) regard it as more potent than *Datura* and use it in instances where extraordinarily difficult divination must be accomplished. The chemical analysis showing the leaves and stems to contain eighty per cent scopolamine in the total assay of alkaloids indicates its potency, which is manifest in excitement, delirium, hallucinations, and coma.

Throughout the central Andes one frequently finds the cactus *Trichocereus*

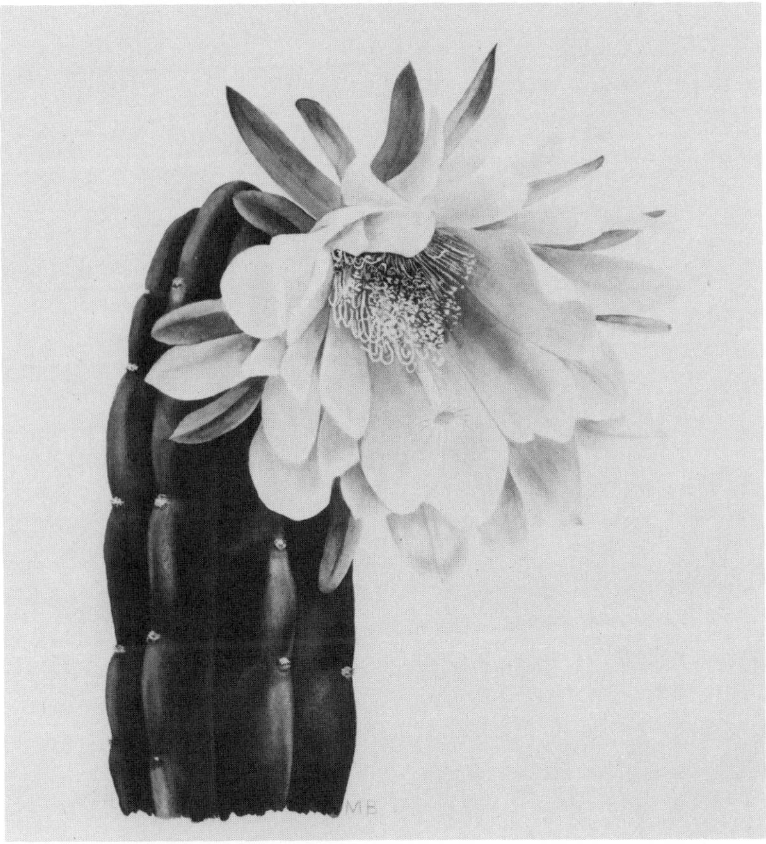

FIG. 65:
Trichocereus pachanoi

pachanoi in cultivation under the name "San Pedro" (Fig. 65). The form of this plant is much like that of *Cereus,* growing to twenty feet in height and comprised of fleshy six- to eight-ribbed branches with few spines. When the latter are present, they are in groups of three to seven. At night the enormous flowers appear at the tip of the branches exuding fragrance from the pale buff outer petals and the reddish inner ones. Although the plant is not closely related to *Lophophora* (peyote), it contains mescaline in the flesh. Throughout eastern Ecuador and Peru the plant is widely cultivated and used to make a hallucinogenic brew called *cimora.* The cactus is stripped of any spines and cut into pieces that are placed into a cauldron with *Neoraimondia macrostibas, Iresine, Isotoma longiflora, Pedilanthus tithymaloides,* and one of the *Daturas.* Water is added to the mixture, and it is allowed to cook for several hours until it has the consistency of pea soup. The brujo or curandero who administers a cup of the brew to his client expects vomiting to follow, and then a period of revelation in which questions may be asked of the intoxicated person or he may be asked to choose among a series of objects, each of which has an individual and collective meaning to the brujo. It may be used in order to take possession of the soul of another. In some instances, it is the brujo or bruja

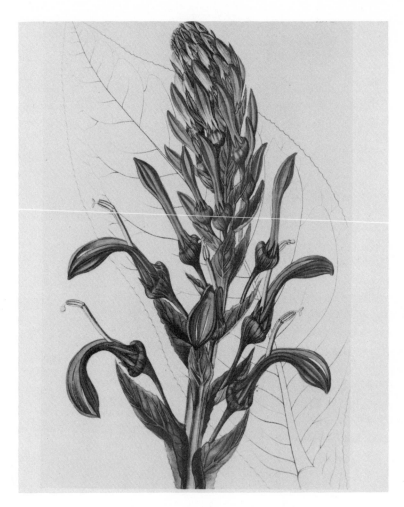

Fig. 66:
Lobelia tupa

who ingests the liquid in order to divine or become prophetic. The antiquity of this ritual use was indicated by Douglas Sharon, who in 1972 wrote of the use of this plant (San Pedro) among folk healers in coastal Peru. Douglas Sharon found images on funeral pottery and painted textiles of Chávin, an Andean civilization dating to 1000 B.C. It reappears later in the ritual art of the Moche and Nazca cultures.

Since mescaline is two per cent of the composition of San Pedro as measured by dry weight, we may expect the effects to be similar to those of peyote unless the admixtures are present that may alter the visions. Dobkin de Rios in 1972 documented a healing ceremony in Peru in which both the folk healer and patient drink a San Pedro brew in order to divine an unknown illness. It would seem that the plant has not been used as a personal inducement to religious contemplation, nor is there evidence for a hedonistic use in Peru or Ecuador. Since the fast-growing cactus has a hardy root system, it is often used throughout the southwestern United States for grafting purposes, in which instances more tender cacti are grown on this plant. A widespread knowledge of the properties of the plant and its current legal status have made it a plant of considerable importance in the United States drug subculture. It is widely available in most cactus nurseries, where it is often sold as an ornamental.

Another plant in wide employ among the Kamsás and Inganos of the Sibundoy, a valley existing at an elevation of 6,700 feet, is *Iochroma fuchsioides (I. umbrosa)* (Pl. 49). Schultes, who has studied this plant in some detail in its habitat, refers to it as a magico-religious narcotic. Formerly the status of use among the people of southern Colombia with respect to this plant was in question. The early studies of Schultes in 1946 had implicated the plant, and later it seemed not to be verified by subsequent investigators. Returning in 1974 Schultes in extensive discourse with a leading Kamsá medicine man found that *Iochroma fuchsioides* leaves were used for difficult diagnoses, divination, and prophecy. The medicine man employing the leaves is often ill for a day or more following his use of the material. Fresh bark and leaves are boiled together and cooled. One to three cupfuls taken over a three-hour period induce hallucinations. It was reported that the plant used to be employed more frequently in earlier days. Known by a variety of popular names such as *borrachera* (intoxicant), the plant is grown by Kamsá medicine men along with *Datura candida* and *Methysticodendron*, indicating something of its status. In chemical analyses thus far, it has not been possible to isolate a known hallucinogen from this red flowered shrub, but it seems that tropane-like alkaloids might be present due to its botanical affinities.

The family Campanulaceae is so large that it has been divided into three subfamilies of which Lobelioideae is one. The distinctions found within this taxon have brought some taxonomists to the view that it should be treated as the family Lobeliaceae. *Tupa* or *tobaco del diablo* is derived from *Lobelia tupa* of the Chilean highlands (Fig. 66). The plant is in no way related to the tobacco of commerce. The tall and highly variable herb has found a place in folk medicine, as the leaves may be pressed to exude a juice reported to be useful in curing toothache. More interesting is the practice among the Mapuche Indians of smoking the leaves for their intoxicating effects that may extend into the realm of hallucinations. We must recall the use of *Lobelia inflata* in North America among the Penobscot Indians of the eastern states. When in 1785 Cutler published his account of this herb and its uses, he noted that the leaves when chewed "produce giddiness and pain of the head, with a trembling agitation." This was the plant that he called "Indian tobacco." While these properties were later ascribed to lobeline, which is also found in *Lobelia tupa*, there may be other yet undiscovered chemicals contributing to the syndrome. In *L. tupa* lobeline, lobelamidine and norlobelamidine have all been reported to be present. Although no one of these may be considered as a hallucinogen, the effect on the Mapuches is much like that reported for the Penobscots. This same family provides *Isotoma longiflora*, an ingredient in *cimora* of the Peruvian Andes and a plant for which we have no satisfactory assay.

In the southern parts of Chile the hillsides support a shrub growing to about three feet in height and known to the natives as *taique* or *chapico*. The botanist recognizes this plant as *Desfontainea spinosa*, based upon its tubular flowers that

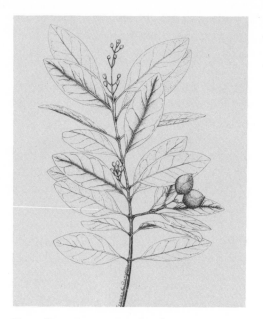
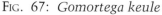
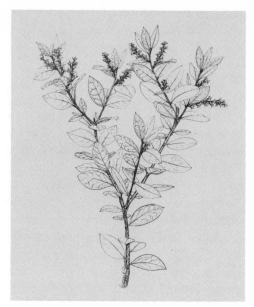

FIG. 67: *Gomortega keule*   FIG. 68: *Pernettya furens*

are bright red tipped with yellow and its holly-like leaves (Pl. 50). *Desfontainea* is the only genus in that family, Desfontainiaceae (formerly included in the Loganiaceae or Potaliaceae), and the variety known as *Hookeri* is that employed as a narcotic. Although it has been known for some time that the leaves of this plant have been used as both a medicant and a narcotic, chemical analyses remain to be carried out.

The Chilean Mapuche Indians also utilize the fresh fruit of the tropical endemic tree *Gomortega keule* of the family Gomortegaceae (Fig. 67). This primitive tree is related to the families Atherospermataceae and Lauraceae and is considered to be primitive among flowering plants. The entire distribution pattern for the tree is within the area of only one hundred square miles. Known as *keule* and *hualhual*, the tree may be found on forested slopes and is easily identified by the shiny evergreen leaves and the small fleshy plum-like fruits that are fragrant and rich in essential oils. It is the fruit oils that are intoxicating, and fresh fruit seems to be more potent than dried. It has been suggested that physiological ammoniation of these oils in the human body may produce an amphetamine-like hallucination, but concrete evidence for this is lacking.

Pernettya furens belongs to the heath family and is common to Chile and surrounding areas (Fig. 68). The fruits are called *huedhued* or *hierba loca*, since eating them causes mental confusion, delirium, and in excess is said to provoke a permanent mental condition that mimics insanity. Some have compared the intoxication to that produced by *Datura*. A related species in Ecuador, *P. parvifolia*, known as *taglli*, is known to cause hallucinations and lack of motor coordination.

122

There is some debate over whether this intoxication is deliberate or accidental, but recently Naranjo has argued for purposeful intoxication. *Pernettya parvifolia* contains andromedotoxin and arbutin, a resin and glucoside respectively. Neither of these may be considered hallucinogenic, but the behavior of the individual who has consumed fruits of these species exhibits every characteristic of one who has experienced a powerful hallucinogen.

In the montane areas of central Chile one infrequently encounters the shrub or small tree *Latua pubiflora*, which was first described in 1888 and also known under the name *L. venemosa* for reason of the venomous nature of the leaves, which contain hyoscyamine and scopolamine (Fig. 69). It is interesting that the natives insist that the fruits also intoxicate, for an analysis of some of the dried fruits revealed no hallucinogens or related compounds. Perhaps fresh fruit might provide different information. In the province of Valdivia, the plant has been known as *latué* and *arbol de los brujos* (tree of the warlocks or sorcerers), for like *Pernettya* it may induce a permanent madness. Those who inhabit this area believe that an accomplished sorcerer can provide a madness of predictable duration according to dosage. Both the preparation and dosages remain carefully guarded secrets in the hands of these malefactors. No cult use apart from the activities of brujos surrounds the plant, and it is generally regarded with fear and suspicion. Given the chemical composition, the hallucination should be much like that from *Datura* or *Hyoscyamus*. It is found only in moist shaded areas, sometimes advancing into meadows at altitudes of about 1,500 feet.

FIG. 69: *Latua pubiflora*   FIG. 70: *Coriaria thymifolia*

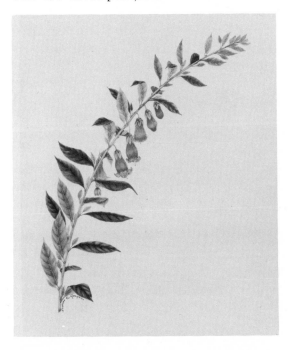

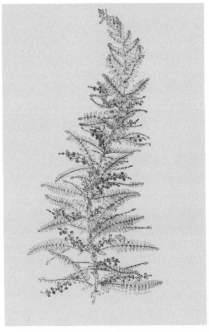

Coriaria thymifolia is found throughout the Ecuadorian Andes as a shrub that is toxic to browsing animals (Fig. 70). It is the only genus in the family Coriariaceae, which is related to the family Sapindaceae. Frond-like leaves of a pinnatifid nature grace the branches, and lateral spikes of tiny flowers are displaced by clusters of small purplish fruits. These fruits when ingested provide sensations of flying. This is thought to be due to catecholic derivatives or an unidentified glucoside. The plant is called *shanshi,* and its use is restricted to sorcerers who indulge in magical flight.

EUROPE AND THE MIDDLE EAST

For all of the herb lore of Europe a few centuries ago, little survives today, and an enumeration of hallucinogenic plants in this area seems comparatively depauperate. I believe that the best explanation for this comes from the famous anthropologist Weston LaBarre of Duke University, who pointed out that the Eurasiatic shamanistic tradition persisted in Western culture in the shamanistic metamorphoses of Zeus, the weather-shaman Hera, the shamanistic trident shared by the brothers Zeus and Poseidon, the animal alter egos of the gods (Apollo—wolf; Zeus—serpent, thunderbird; Artemis—stag; Athena—owl, snake; Dionysus—bull; etc.). Even the gods had their oracles: Zeus at Olympus and Apollo at Delphi. Did the Delphic Oracle have hallucinogens in the censer while she reposed on her three-legged stool? By what magic did Circe change men into swine? What was the odorous ambrosia of the gods? How does one explain the potency of the seed cake of Ceres? In one brilliantly laconic statement, LaBarre answers many of these questions: "And when the anthropomorphic God dies, we have left the impersonal forces of science." As Harner pointed out in 1973, the additional factor of the Church considering shamanic practices and the utilization of hallucinogens to be heretic led to the abolition of such practices, obscuring much of the Western tradition. Thus the traditions of shamanic witchcraft are regarded by some scholars as a fiction created by the Church, especially during the Inquisition. We must remember that early Western civilization had its roots in a strong Eurasian shamanistic background, and this remains reflected in our mythology. Displacement of these traditions has left only hints of ritualistic practices, which were doubtless as varied and bizarre as those found among aboriginal peoples of today. By culling mythology, witchcraft, and folk medicine traditions from European lore, we may find an even greater number of psychoactive plants that have been employed in the Old World as compared to the New World traditions.

Instead of centering our attention solely on aboriginal cultures and the remnants of defunct New World cultures, perhaps we need to relearn the roots of our own shamanistic traditions and find the specific plants that were associated with that which is now taken to be myth and legend. A reinvestigation of the mystical Old World and its supernatural traditions is sorely needed.

Syrian rue is a name used to describe a woody perennial shrub found growing in dry areas of the Mediterranean, in northern India, Mongolia, and Manchuria. Known to botanists as *Peganum harmala* of the family Zygophyllaceae, it is famous for its use in producing the dye called "Turkish red," which is obtained from the abundant

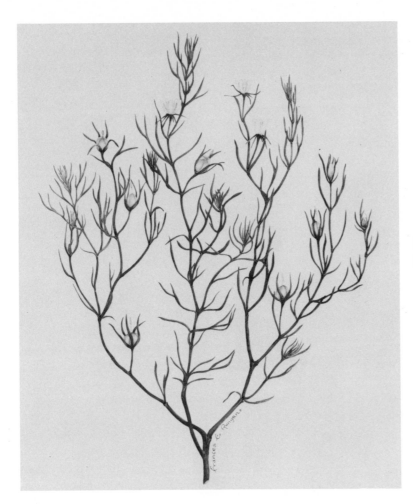

Fig. 71:
Peganum harmala

seed (Fig. 71). It is used to produce color characteristic of all of the Iranian and Turkish carpets. Dioscorides spoke of this plant in his famous codex *(Codex Vindobonensis)* of the first century. The written history of this plant extends over a thousand years. In Egypt the oil from this seed is sold as *zit-el-harmel* and has the reputation of being an aphrodisiac. Medicinal uses extend to its use in treating diseases of the eyes, as a vermifuge, soporific, lactogogue, etc. The seed is widely known as a narcotic, and analyses reveal harmaline, harmalol, and harmine. Harmine is now in use in research on mental disease, encephalitis, and inflammation of the brain. Small doses are stimulating to the brain and reportedly are therapeutic, but in excess harmine depresses the central nervous system. During the Second World War, Nazi "scientists" used harmine to advantage as a truth serum. In reality there is no truth serum, but an alteration in thresholds of consciousness may make a person loquacious. A crude preparation of the seed is more effective than any extract because of the presence of related indoles. The Douvans of Bokhara used to inhale the smoke of burning *Peganum harmala* seed and became quite exuberant,

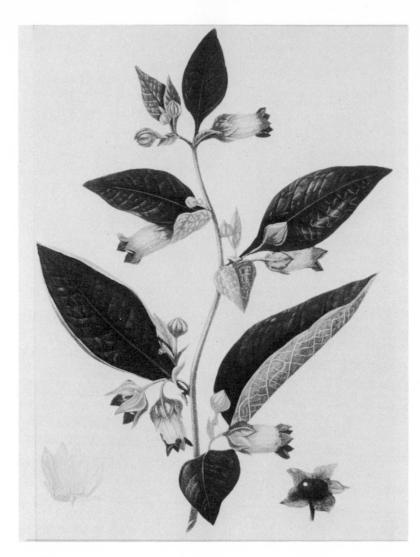

F<small>IG</small>. 72:
Atropa belladonna

much in the manner of the people of South America using *caapi*, which has the same class of chemicals. This is one of the few clues as to possible historical uses in a shamanic context, and at this time no one has done any thorough research on it.

Notable among the European herbs used to induce hallucinations is the enchanter's nightshade or *Atropa belladonna* (Fig. 72). Known as devil's herb, apples of Sodom, and deadly nightshade, this solanaceous plant is said to be tended by the devil himself, who nightly looks after this plant except on Walpurgis night, when he retires to the mountains to prepare for the witches' sabbath. At such a time the herb may metamorphose into an enchantress lovely to behold, but deadly in the viewing. Another tradition relates that Roman priests would drink an infusion of belladonna before appealing to Bellona, goddess of war. *Atropa* is derived from the name of one of the Greek Parcae, *Atropos*, who was believed to be responsible for measuring out the thread of a man's life at the time he was born. The ancient Norse knew the plant as *dwale*, meaning trance, stupor, or sleep.

In the Bacchanalian orgies a spiked wine was drunk, which purportedly contained belladonna, mandrake root, and other narcotic adulterants; such additives would explain the frenzy and hysteria that are not characteristic of wine intoxication, and yet figure prominently into the *sparagmos* of the maenads or bacchantes who tore apart living animals and children. *Atropa* also figures into medieval witches' brews and flying ointments along with henbane, mandrake, and the fat of a stillborn child. The mixture was used as an ointment rubbed onto the body or introduced via the mucous membranes of the vaginal labia. This practice is associated with the witch on her "anointed" broomstick.

Bergamo, who wrote about 1470–71, left an unpublished manuscript, now in the Bibliothèque National, Paris, which was translated by Hansen in 1901. In this we find an account of witches who "anoint a staff and ride on it to the appointed place or anoint themselves under the arms and in other hairy places. . . ." Many women were accused of participating in witchcraft in such a manner. Spina in 1523 told of the Inquisition in the diocese of Como, which was carried out in the walled city of Lugano. A wife of a notary of the Inquisition was accused of being a witch and a sorceress. Her husband sought after her when she was absent on Good Friday. He finally encountered her in the pigsty. "There he found her naked in some corner, displaying her genitals, completely unconscious and smeared with the excrement of pigs." She confessed to having made the witch's journey and drowned herself before she could be burned.

Andrés Laguna, physician to Pope Julius III, in 1545 gave an account of seizing from a married couple accused of being a witch and a warlock, a jar half-filled with an unguent he determined to be nightshade, hemlock, henbane (*Hyoscyamus niger*, Fig. 73), and mandrake. Being a physician, he tested his find on the wife of a hangman in the city of Metz. Since the woman suffered from insomnia, Laguna decided to test the baneful unguent, anointing the woman "from head to toe." She fell into a deep sleep for thirty-six hours. Since she had had lascivious and unfaithful imaginations during this period, Laguna concluded that such potions corrupt the memory, leading to the firm belief by the anointed ones that they have done all that they dreamt in a waking state.

Giovanni Battista Porta in 1562 wrote a book on *Natural Magic* in which he elucidated the contents of witch's salve, which he reports he gleaned from speaking with and observing witches. The revelation was as follows (botanical identifications in parentheses are my own): "they mix eleoselinum, aconite (*Aconitum napellus* root), poplar branches (*Poplus* tree buds provide a lipid balm as a matrix in which to retain the active principals), and soot. Or sometimes sium (*Helossciadium nodiflorum*, an umbel known as sion and marshwort), common acorum (*Acorus calamus* whose rhizome oils are known to be narcotic), the blood of a bat, sleep-inducing nightshade *(Atropa belladonna)*, and oil." All of this was mixed with boy's fat that had been boiled in a copper kettle and strained. After describing the effects on a self-professed witch who stripped before him and anointed herself thoroughly with the mixture, he cautions melancholics who experiment with the salve, "since their nature is chill and cold nothing very much happens to them from the warming-up methods of witches." Several twentieth-century experimenters have followed the receipt of Porta and experienced the strange visions. Obviously the boy's fat, soot, and bat blood are unnecessary. It should be mentioned that *Aconitum napellus* is a deadly root, and the popular name wolfbane derives from its use in poisoning wolves.

The visions of flying and the common belief of being transformed into one or more of several animals may well explain, in part, the animal alter ego of the shaman. It also sheds light on the vampire (witches were invariably accused of sucking blood), and even the werewolf syndrome. In a book by Porta in 1589 he gives a specific formula for making a man believe that he is transformed into a bird or a beast: henbane, mandrake, stramonium, or *Solanum manicum*, and belladonna. Such a combination would do much to explain lycanthropy. Paulus Aegineta, a

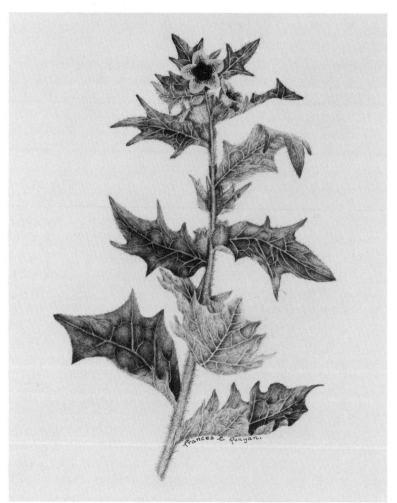

FIG. 73:
Hyoscyamus niger

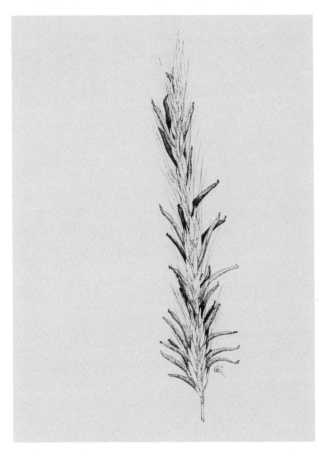

Greek writing of lycanthropy in the fourth to seventh centuries, states that in addition to imitating wolves and lingering about sepulchres, they are recognized by their pale flesh, feeble vision, parched mouth, and ulcerations of the legs from falling a great deal. The formula presented by Porta would produce just such effects due to the abundance of hyoscyamine, scopolamine, and atropine. Thus, there is a botanical, historical, chemical, physiological, and psychological basis for belief in witches, warlocks, sorcerers, vampires, werewolves, and just about every other implausible figure in history. A fine exposition of the role of hallucinogens in European witchcraft was presented by Michael Harner in 1973.

An overview of hallucinogens in Europe would not be complete without an account of "Saint Anthony's Fire," a disease that led its victims on a flight to Egypt to seek help at the shrine of St. Anthony, who had founded an order to care for those afflicted by "Holy Fire." Since the Middle Ages, famine has usually resulted from failure of the staple grain crops upon which most civilizations depend. In times of severe shortage, every ounce of grain becomes a precious commodity, and diseased crops that are usually rejected are ravenously consumed. A peculiar dark grain which the French dubbed *argot*, referring to a spur, became transliterated to ergot.

This is the result of individual grains becoming parasitized during their development by the fungus *Claviceps purpurea* (Fig. 74). Once the grain contacts the spore, it is soon replaced by the fungal body that develops on it producing a dark purple-brown grain-like structure that is about a centimeter in length and furrowed, resembling the normal grain. It has been estimated that a crop infected with less than one per cent of ergot is sufficient to cause an outbreak of the plague known as *ergotisme* or ergotism. Desperate harvesting in famine years resulted in the contamination of bread so that entire villages would fall prey to the disease, which led to the speculation that such villages were possessed of the Devil and suffering in his eternal fires. Pregnant women would spontaneously abort, others would suffer strange delusions and feel their bodies being consumed by flames. After a time, the afflicted would exhibit gangrenous limbs and a number would die. The Order of Saint Anthony, who is easily recognized by his companion the pig, would care for these victims. Until the seventeenth century, a number of these orders exhibited the fallen limbs of their patients as a testimonial to the numbers of afflicted who had been treated.

Midwives soon learned the source of this evil and employed grains of ergot in their practices. They found that five to nine of the ergot grains could be administered to hasten difficult births without any post-parturition hemorrhage. Later ergot was to find its way into diverse medical practices. One of the most popular contemporary uses is to combine the ergot with caffeine to constrict dialated capillaries in instances of migraine headaches. Unfortunately, not all migraines are caused by vasodilation and in some instances the medicine is of no avail.

In 1906 ergotoxine was isolated as the first alkaloid to be derived from this peculiar ascomycete. Later, in 1920, ergotamine and ergotaminine were identified, and subsequently close to a dozen other alkaloids have been extracted and identified. Ergometrine (ergonovine) is the component responsible for hemostatic action in the uterus. Isoergine (isolysergic acid) seems to induce apathy and mental depression. Both elymoclavine and lysergol are central nervous system stimulants. The action of d-lysergic acid is that of somnolence and a clouding of consciousness. In 1938 Albert Hofmann of the Sandoz Laboratories synthesized d-lysergic acid diethylamide, which is better known under the initials LSD. The hallucinogenic activity was demonstrated in 1943, for this the most powerful of hallucinogens. In man the effective oral dose of LSD is 0.05 mg. It seems unfortunate that much of the research conducted to determine the possible injurious effects of this hallucinogen has involved massive doses injected in the peritoneal cavity of rodents.

The accounts recorded by Hofmann in April of 1943 are as revealing as any with respect to the action on the human body. After an initial ingestion of what he suspected to be LSD-25, for reason of its being the twenty-fifth isolate in the lysergic acid series, he put the material aside for a week. Then, under controlled conditions he took an oral dose of one-quarter of a milligram of LSD, a large dose for a human, and experienced six hours of spectacular and dramatic visionary experiences involving new and unexperienced levels of consciousness. Since this time, the drug LSD has provoked more controversy than any other. Those who argue that the drug may precipitate a psychosis are confronted with the dilemma of not being able to ascertain how many of these individuals would have become psychotic in the absence of LSD. Those who argue for its safety must take into account the unpredictable behavior of the participant. The belief that one has the ability to soar may be tested. Flying and levitation are not uncommon to this experience.

While a number of psychiatrists have conducted LSD therapy with some interesting results, there are behavioral patterns that even these neo-shamans cannot predict. In one individual the same dosage has different effects at different times. The widest testing programs were carried out as covert activities of the CIA and the Pentagon in cooperation with the U.S. Army. Over a twelve-year period individuals were being subjected to LSD experimentation, without the drug being identified to the individuals in many instances. This was during a period when civilian medical research was being restricted and curtailed. The Army sought Hofmann for a process whereby they might produce many kilograms of the material. During this period the drug remained illegal, and the penalties for conviction were harsh. A New York *Times* exposé of August 1, 1975, uncovered the aforementioned, making it obvious that the military sought the material as an element in chemical warfare, for the amounts sought would have easily "turned on" a city the size of greater Los Angeles! All of this was carried out while information suggesting chromosomal damage, spontaneous abortion, permanent psychoses, and other disasters resulting from the drug was being systematically fed to the public.

The appearance of a new hallucinogen regularly arouses a kind of moral indignation among the public. New pleasures are always the stimulus for the alteration of existing moral values, so that judgements are rarely rational and have a tendency to reflect fear, confusion, and uninformed moral pronouncements. It is only after some experimentation that drug abuse may be properly defined, unless it is accepted that all drug use constitutes abuse. Laws surrounding LSD use have been based more on panic and power than on research data. None of this suggests that LSD is safe or is not; it does serve to point up the dilemma of the Western world that has lost its shamanism and has not successfully supplanted it with religion. There is every reason to believe that man still requires some respite from his physical and psychological woes and the freedom to step beyond himself. Control by legislation has not historically been of any success.

Lewis Lewin said "man has a passionate desire to flee from the monotony of everyday life." I think that we might append to this the *fear* of everyday life as well. In an age of great uncertainty and great despair, it is understandable that man will attempt to seek other realms, to reach out beyond the impersonal forces of both science and technology to experience a world created both from without and from within. *Induced* personal mysticism is not new to the world, and it is not likely to disappear. Since man first strayed from the non-nutritive aspects of the plant world and explored the realms of consciousness within himself, he has never departed from these forays. Withholding judgment, it is safe to say that man has, and always will attempt to explore his diverse states of consciousness. This renewed broad interest in experimenting with the selves within may best characterize the past several decades of this century as reviewed by some future historian.

STIMULANTS

"Let us dream of evanescence,
and linger in the beautiful
foolishness of things."

Okakura-Kakuzo
The Book of Tea

"Excitantia" is the term used by Lewin to describe drugs that stimulate the nervous system. Some of these stimulants have played a role in the development of entire civilizations, others have histories rooted in debauchery and plunder, still others menace populations with the threat of disease. Many of us would find it difficult to make it through a day without one or more of these "analeptics." Indeed, the tea or coffee break is one of the few rituals still widely practiced by English and Americans. Most stimulants are derived from botanical sources and have histories that are best classified in accord with their properties—"excitantia." A review of botanical sources of analeptics associated with major civilizations will reveal the ways in which man has employed these drugs.

Tea is first mentioned in the Chinese dictionary of Kuo P'o, which appeared in A.D. 350. Earlier attributions are incorrect. "Cha" was the name used then and still used in China. Although our first records are from China, tea grows as a native only in northern Thailand, East Burma, Assam, Yunnan, upper Indo-China, and parts of India. Tea is in the same genus as the horticultural *Camellia.* Formerly known as *Thea sinensis* (literally, tea of China), it is properly called *Camellia thea* (Fig. 75).

Under varying conditions of cultivation, tea leaves will develop distinctive flavors. Even leaves on the same plant vary in quality, and only immature leaves are suitable for use in choice tea. Buds and the few terminal leaves produce teas of a quality seldom encountered in domestic markets. An expert can distinguish over a hundred grades of tea from this single species. Of course, the treatment which follows harvesting imparts much of the flavor. Black tea is the result of "withering" the leaves in the sun and then crushing them slightly so that some of the cells are broken, releasing enzymes that will ferment the leaves and extract the tannins. At a critical moment in fermentation the leaves are "fired" at 200 degrees Fahrenheit to end the process. Green tea differs in that the fermentation is restricted. Oolong tea differs from the other two in being "withered" for only a brief time and being fired for only a few moments at 400 degrees Fahrenheit.

In addition to caffeine, which acts as a mild stimulant to the cerebral cortex, tea contains theophylline, which causes dilation of the coronary artery supplying the heart. These xanthines in moderate doses pose no threat to the individual with normal metabolism, but there have been critics of this "addiction." Like most stimulants, the addiction is a psychological state; rather than having a physiological basis, it is habituating. Since the per capita consumption of tea in England is over ten pounds annually, ten cups per day is not unusual. Tea contains about one and one half grains of caffeine per cup, about one half of the recommended medical dosage. In 1952 a medical member of the House of Commons spoke out against excesses in tea drinking. In his words, such individuals "pose before us as virtuous people, forgetting that they are the truest types of drug addicts." Given the American penchant for prohibition, it should surprise us that no proposal restricting the drinking of tea has been introduced into our legislation.

Tea is, by dry weight, 4.5 per cent caffeine and theophylline, the latter known also as theocin or dimethylxanthine. Any consumption in excess of five cups of tea per day constitutes a form of drug abuse. Louis Lewin recorded instances in which a man who drank thirty cups of tea per day suffered anemia, suffocation, and hallucinations. Teaism is characterized by gastric disorders, pale or yellow skin,

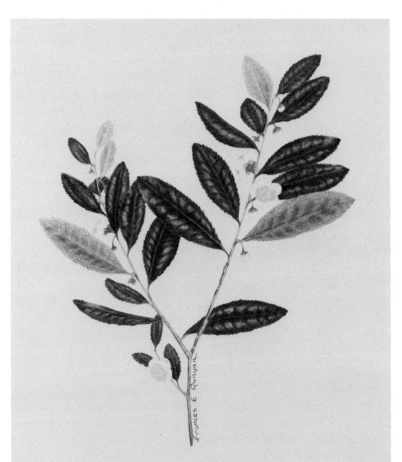

FIG. 75:
*Camellia thea
(Thea sinensis)*

nervous disorders, hypochondria, sight disturbances, weakening of memory, liver malfunction, and chromosomal breakage. The effects on the kidneys may result in acute nephritis.

While we usually presume tea consumption to be in the form of hot or iced tea or perhaps as a flavoring agent in ice cream, there was a mode of consumption in England no longer encountered. Haysan tea was made into cigarettes that were particularly favored by women in the first quarter of this century. The xanthines present pass into the smoke and enter the circulatory system in the lungs. The response in a heavy smoker was nervousness, trembling, heart palpations, and a general restlessness.

If all of this were not enough to frighten the tea drinker, recent reports indicate that old tea leaves that are used to make the less expensive brands of tea, especially those popularly marketed in the United States, are high in tannins. Tannins accumulate in mature leaves as metabolic byproducts and are absent in the very young shoots and small leaves that are used to produce fine teas such as the costly silverpoint. Stomach cancer in experimental animals has been induced through the introduction of excessive amounts of tannins.

Somewhere between the praise of Okakura-Kakuzo and the condemnation of those who have witnessed the effects of tea abuse is the happy middle ground of moderation. A few cups of choice tea that is finely brewed can be an extremely pleasant experience that is not fraught with the dangers inherent in abuse.

Before leaving the subject of tea, it is worthwile recounting some of the rather bizarre uses in Tibet. Weary horses and mules are given large vessels of tea to increase their capacity to work. Mules are said to be seen gamboling about like colts as a result of their tea rations. Equally interesting is the use of tea as a measure of distance, for tea, as we will see later with cocoa, is used as a measure of time. The distance between villages is accounted for in terms of the number of cups of tea necessary to sustain the person traveling that route. It has been ascertained that three cups of tea is equal to eight kilometers. Mongolians have had the most interesting practice of brewing tea ever recorded. Inferior tea leaves that would normally be discarded are compressed into flat cakes known as "tea tiles." These are held together by first mixing the leaves with yak feces and kneading the two together. The dried "tea tiles" may be used at any later date by breaking off a piece and boiling it with water to which butter or yak fat has been added. Certainly this ceremony is not allied to the Chinese practice of reducing the dried green leaves to a powder and whipping this into boiling salted water. Perhaps to the Mongolian our contemporary practice of using fermented black teas mixed with all manner of spice and citrus rinds as well as milk and sugar would seem just as bizarre as their dung and fat tea.

Avicenna, the famous Arabian philospher and physician (980–1037), was one of the first to write about coffee. Because of this Arabian record, Linnaeus, the Swedish botanist of the eighteenth century, named the plant *Coffea arabica* (Pl. 51). Evidence is rather conclusive that the home of coffee is Ethiopia. In 1601 Anthony Sherley introduced *Kahveh* into England, and William Parry wrote of it using the contemporary spelling "coffee," which he originated. So popular was the beverage, that coffeehouses spread rapidly throughout Europe and by 1689 even Boston had its "café." Demands for the seed of *Coffea arabica* were so great that the world powers began to establish the plants in their colonies. Not until the eighteenth century did South America become a center of cultivation. Now two-thirds of the world's supply of coffee comes from São Paulo, Brazil, in the form of 132-pound bags; forty million such bags supply the world's annual requirements.

Berries of the coffee plant look very like our cranberries, and each fruit contains two seeds that when dried, aged, roasted, and ground, form the coffee of commerce. These seeds contain only about one per cent caffeine which, when infused, gives the weary a lift through a direct effect on the cortex of the brain. While numerous other sources of caffeine are available, Americans prefer coffee beans, consuming seventeen pounds annually on a per capita basis.

Inherent in the use of coffee are the same perils found in drinking excessive amounts of tea. The organic acids are likely to create stomach and intestinal disturbances. It was coffee that was said to have ruined the stomach of the French minister, Colbert. Because of the early recognition of the effect of coffee in making the populace excessively loquacious, in 1511 edicts against it were issued in several European countries. The Prince of Waldeck by the grace of God offered a reward of ten thalers to anyone who would give over the name of a coffee drinker. By 1777 the Prince-Bishop Wilhelm of Paderborn announced that coffee drinking was the privilege of aristocracy and the clergy, but not suitable for the middle class or peasants, and prohibition among them was continued. It was no great deprivation, for the ordinary man could hardly afford the price of coffee. Punishment for coffee offenses usually consisted of a public beating. This was generally supplanted by heavy taxation.

It is interesting to note that when prohibition was instituted in the United States, the consumption of coffee, tea, and cocaine soared. Individuals simply do not abstain, they substitute the drug of choice for another that is more readily available.

Coffee was used by monks for reason of remaining alert during the protracted evening masses and vespers. A more important aspect of this use derives from the early report of Olearius, who stated that the Persians drank coffee to "sterilize their natures and extinguish carnal desires." It was said that the wife of a sultan who had been sexually ignored, watching a stallion being castrated, suggested that it would be better to give the animal coffee, for this, she asserted, had deprived her husband of his manhood. The very opposite is true, for coffee is a uro-genital stimulant. Princess Liselotte of Orlean in writing to one of her sisters suggested that coffee was suitable for Catholic priests who are not allowed to marry and must remain chaste. Since her husband, Regent Philip II, was given to coffee and known to all but his wife for "dissipation," it is not so surprising a statement.

The great writer Goethe believed that the coffee with milk that he took after meals gave him a sad and melancholic disposition as well as paralyzing his intestines, which in turn generated anxiety. These peculiar belief systems must be separated from the true attributes of coffee. Fortunately, the coffee drinker of today may have his coffee with the organic acids removed or the xanthines absent or both. Despite all of the refined means of processing coffee, there is no doubt in the mind of

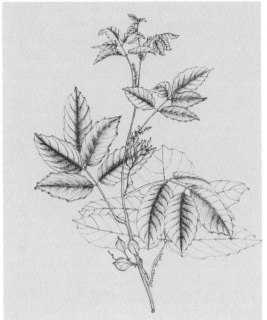

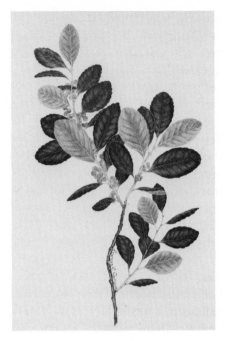

FIG. 76: *Paullinia cupana*   FIG. 77: *Ilex paraguayensis*

the lover of coffee that the finest preparation comes from the freshly roasted and ground beans prepared with the ingenious expresso machine that extracts the essence from the fragrant seed. Neither extravagant prices for coffee nor information on the harmful effects has had any influence on the ever-increasing demand for coffee throughout most of the world.

In October of each year, the Manes and Manduru Kus of the lower and middle Tapajós in the Amazon collect seeds of a woody liana, *Paullinia cupana* (Fig. 76). These seeds mold quite easily, so they are ground and mixed with cassava flour, from the root of *Manihot esculenta,* and water to form a chocolate-colored paste. *Guarana* paste is shaped into cylinders that are baked slowly over wood fires until they are as hard as stone. Dried *guarana* sticks are shipped to Bolivia and Matto Grosso where they are grated on the tongue of a piraracu, a large fish of the Amazon. One-half teaspoon of *guarana* shavings in a cup of sweetened hot or cold water is as indispensable to these people as is our morning cup of coffee—and a lot more potent, for *guarana* contains about five per cent caffeine. Related species of *Paullinia* contain as much as three per cent caffeien in their bark, and to the Indian of the Colombian Putumayo *yopo* squeezed from the bark of *Paullinia yopo* is his entire sustenance until noon each day. Ritualistically, the Indians of this area avoid food before midday, and this strong stimulant stays fatigue and hunger. *Paullinia cupana* is thought to have been in cultivation for over thousands of years, whereas coffee was not introduced into Brazil until 1774.

In the mountains of southern Brazil, Paraguay, and Argentina a small tree or evergreen shrub, *Ilex paraguayensis,* known to the Indians as maté yerba, was used as a stimulant for centuries before the Conquest (Fig. 77). This shrub, with its deep-green leaves and white flowers, bears a striking resemblance to tea, and when in fruit, somewhat resembles coffee. Branches from the tips of the shrub are cut before the leaves have matured (at maturity they may be five inches in length) and are toasted over open fires to vaporize resins and reduce moisture content; finally, they are threshed and sifted to remove twigs. Aging of the toasted leaves helps develop both the flavor and the aroma. Since the appearance of the conquistadors, the popularity of maté spread rapidly, and it became known as Jesuit tea in many areas. Although most of the two hundred thousand tons produced annually comes from plants growing in the wild, plantations in Brazil are now growing a considerable acreage of maté. Two-thirds of the annual harvest is consumed in Argentina, and little appears in the United States. Maté is used to flavor some soft drinks.

Maté grows rapidly and can produce a crop from seed after one year's growth. It has a second advantage in not requiring extensive cultivation. The leaves of older plants are usually preferred, for they contain about 0.5 per cent to over 1 per cent caffeine. In addition to this stimulant, there are some vitamins and volatile oils giving the beverage a characteristic aroma. While the beverage is frequently prepared much like tea, in the more primitive areas the leaves are carried in a horn or gourd, and cold water is poured over them. After steeping the leaves in the water, a *bombilla,* or hollow tube of silver, brass, or straw terminating in a perforated bowl, is immersed in the *cuya* containing maté. Among the Guarani Indians, the bowl of this greenish infusion is ceremonially passed around a group, and when the liquid is exhausted, water may be poured over the leaves to renew the decoction. Such were the "tea parties" held in the Americas long before Europeans entertained the idea of a New World.

"Food of the gods" was the description of cocoa that Doña Marina gave Cortes when he landed in the Yucatan peninsula in the year 1519. Having defeated the Maya Indians who inhabited the region, Cortes was given nineteen girls as loot from this conquest; records indicate that Cortes hardly considered them as treasures. Among them, however, was the beautiful princess Doña Marina, who spoke both the language of the Mayas and that of the Aztecs. After she perfected her Spanish, Cortes used her as an interpreter during the subsequent Spanish conquests. It was through Doña Marina, who had by this time been mistress to Cortes and wife to one of his captains, that Cortes found the bitter beverage that was consumed only by Montezuma and his lords. Given the splendor of the riches taken from this Aztec king, Cortes was ready to believe almost anything; thus, when the aging Montezuma was seen drinking a concoction of raw cacao beans ground with red pepper and bitter herbs before going to a harem of beautiful women, Cortes was understandably curious. Doña Marina assured Cortes that the mixture drunk from a golden vessel was a potent aphrodisiac. Thousands of the small plants from which the cocoa was derived were ordered planted by Cortes so that Europe might know the joys residing in this tiny bean. Having gained the ultimate knowledge, Cortes dealt the Aztecs a final blow, the regicide of 1520.

Native to the Amazon Valley, the tree had been brought to Mexico centuries before the entry of Cortes. Seeds from the pulp of this large orange fruit were used by the Indians as currency before and after the Conquest. In spite of the reputation of *chocolatl* (the Aztec term) as an aphrodisiac, nuns in a cloister at Chiapas in 1550 discovered that when the powdered seed was mixed with vanilla and sugar, a delicious beverage resulted. So popular was this drink that the ladies had their maids bring the brew to them to drink during mass at the cathedral. When the Bishop spoke out against this practice, the ladies, who maintained that *chocolatl* "overcomes weakness of the stomach," removed themselves to the cloister church to join the nuns in this harmless pastime. Actually, there are no aphrodisiac properties, only a mild stimulation from the alkaloid theobromine which is almost identical to caffeine.

Linnaeus did not ignore the story of Montezuma, for when he christened the tree with the generic epithet *Theobroma*, he repeated in Greek the words of Doña Marina, "food of the gods." Each *Theobroma cacao* tree bears thousands of tiny yellow flowers, not on the twigs, but arising directly from the trunk and older branches. Only a few dozen of these ever develop into the obovate fruits containing a pulpy white mucilage in which are to be found the cacao beans. (Fig. 78). After fermenting and cleaning, the beans, which are about the size of lima beans, are roasted and the husk is removed by crushing. Cocoa and chocolate are both derived from this residue, the only difference being that cocoa results from the removal of most of the natural oil in the bean, whereas chocolate is the residue plus fortification through the addition of the oils extracted in cocoa manufacture. In both cases sugar is added and sometimes milk or arrowroot. An innocent confection born out of conquest, myth, and plunder is produced annually from eight hundred thousand tons of cacao beans. Most of the crop is produced in Nigeria and Ghana, but a substantial portion comes from Brazil. More recently Nicaragua and Costa Rica have planted this crop. Until 1910 plantations in Venezuela, Ecuador, Brazil, and São Thomé (off the coast of Africa) were run by slave labor. Since then, this crop, like coffee, has financed the extensive spread of civilization in these areas.

Almost as popular as coffee are the cola drinks, yet few people consider them stimulants. Native to tropical western Africa, *Cola nitida* (cf. *C. acuminata*) has been introduced to various parts of the world because of the kola nut, which yields two per cent caffeine by weight and has a pleasant flavor (Fig. 79). Inside the star-shaped fruits, which are about ten centimeters long, there are eight reddish to white seeds. Natives of Africa and Jamaica chew the seeds of this tree fresh or boil them to form a beverage inhibiting fatigue and hunger. Nearly one hundred tons of these dried seeds are imported into the United States every year to be used primarily in cola drinks.

Khunu, god of snow, thunder, and lightning, was angered by chiefs of the Yunga who had allowed their people to burn his forests and blacken his temples—the Illimani and the Mururata snow-capped peaks. Banishment from the capital and Lake Titicaca was the price of this outrage. Leading a nomadic existence cut off from their *mallcos* (supreme chiefs), the Yunga leaders roamed about the mountains. Almost dead from lack of water and fatigue, they chanced upon coca leaves. Upon

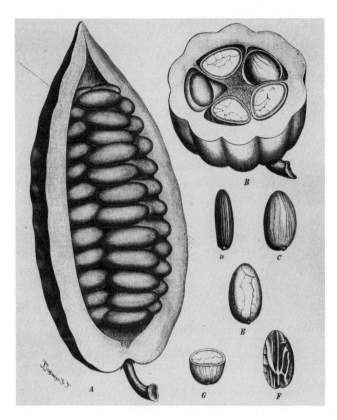

FIG. 78:
Theobroma cacao

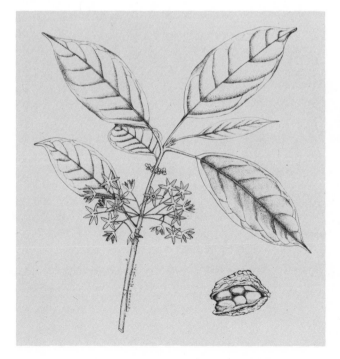

FIG. 79:
Cola nitida

139

chewing these they were able to cross the treacherous mountains to Tiahuanaco without suffering from mountain sickness. This is one of the several legends used to explain the miraculous plant *Erythroxylum coca* (Pl. 52). Coca originated in Bolivia in the region of Machu Yunga (formerly High Peru). The Arawaks learned the practice of coca chewing from their conquerors, the Chibchas, who migrated across the Andes. These two tribes and the Quetchuas originated the cultivation of *Erythroxylum*, a practice that spread to Central America, the West Indies, and the northern part of South America.

Mayta-Capac (A.D. 1230) and Rocca, his successor who died in 1315, are the two Incas responsible for the wide distribution of *Erythroxylum*, for they regarded coca as a divinity to be venerated and worshipped. By the end of the fourteenth century this sacred plant was in widespread use among the Incas. It is a most attractive woody shrub bearing simple obovate bright-green leaves and brilliant red berries. *Coquero* is a name applied to the male chewer of coca leaves; actually, chewing is a misnomer, for the *chique* or quid is sucked rather than chewed. Repeated wedging of the quid between teeth and cheek leads eventually to a deformed cheek (Fig. 80).

Just as the African women slaves chewed kola nuts to relieve hunger and fatigue, Andean porters and guides chew the leaves of *Erythroxylum coca*. Coca is the only source of cocaine, a stimulant that has an almost immediate action on the higher levels of the brain, giving the user a sense of boundless energy and freedom

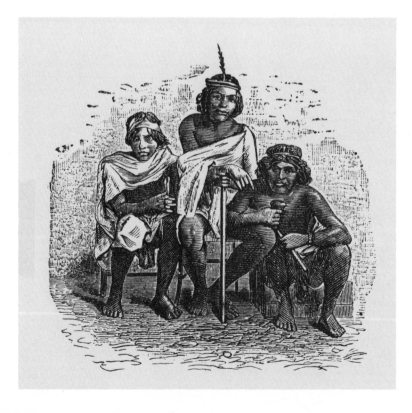

FIG. 80:
Coca chewers
(From Mariani)

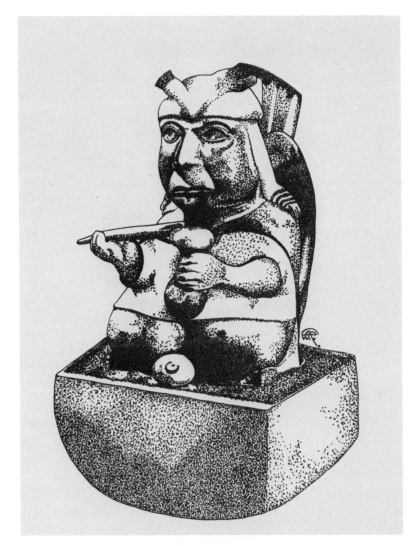

FIG. 81: Andean stone figure of a man with a popóro

from fatigue. It was one of the basic ingredients of Coca-Cola, together with *Cola nitida*, until 1904 when the United States courts ruled against its use. Now the leaves minus cocaine are still used as a flavoring agent. Coca leaves were employed centuries before Pizarro conquered Peru. Grave sites indicate that the pattern of use has not changed (Fig. 81). Every mature Indian has a vicuña bag used to carry the dried leaves, a small block of lime from quinoa ash *(llipta)* inside a gourd *(popóro)*, and a stick for extracting the alkali from the gourd (Fig. 82). To the wad of leaves being chewed, every so often a bit of lime is added; the extracted cocaine acts directly on the central nervous system to relieve the pangs of hunger and fatigue. In the two ounces of dried leaves that an Indian consumes in a day, there are approximately 0.7 grains of cocaine. Doses of this size are never fatal or addictive. In

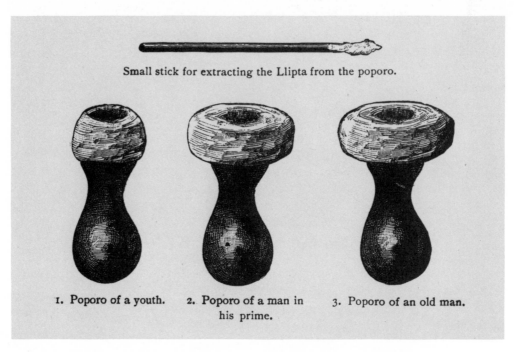

Small stick for extracting the Llipta from the poporo.

1. Poporo of a youth. 2. Poporo of a man in his prime. 3. Poporo of an old man.

FIG. 82: Poporos and llipta

the sixteenth century the Spaniards were extracting gold from the Potosi mines by Inca slave labor, relying upon coca to keep the workers going. In the twentieth century the tradition persists in Bolivia, where American mining is accomplished by laborers who, for reason of almost non-existent wages, must rely on coca.

An Italian physician, Angelo Mariani, amassed a fortune in the nineteenth century by adding coca to wine and selling it under the name "Vin Mariani," and also in a more potent form as a liquor. Both were sold as anesthetics and analgesics with further claims as to their efficacy in curing stomachitis, gingivitis, and gastric disturbances. The argument must have been convincing, for Mariani's customers included such figures as Sarah Bernhardt and Pope Leo XIII. Of the twenty-eight million pounds produced annually, most is consumed in South America.

Coca is now one of the primary drugs used in the wealthy drug subcultures. The cost of "coke" makes it prohibitive for those on a low budget. This accounts for the high frequency of "cut" material appearing when samples of street coca are analyzed by reputable laboratories. Surrogate crystals are frequently sold as cocaine, and they consist of lactose, table sugar, ground glass, and a host of other chemicals. The naive purchaser may simply trust the seller and, depending on the chemical, may become simply another statistic in the coroner's office. More sophisticated users either send the sample to a reputable laboratory for an anonymous analysis or they will use one of the testing kits obtained from "head shops." The latter range from useless color reagents to *fairly* reliable equipment that determines the specific melting point of the sample in question. None of these identifies unknowns.

Coca represents one of the few drugs still involved in a sort of ritual use in Western civilization. A "line" of "coke" is run across a paper bill and snorted into one nostril. A more elaborate ritual involves the use of a minuscule spoon, frequently worn as ornamental jewelry around the neck, which is filled with the white crystal and brought to the nostril for inhalation. The nature of this ritual seems bizarre when one considers that the drug is less efficacious when inhaled than when ingested, so that it is not a ritual based upon reason. The popularity of the drug is attested to by the numerous fine jewelry stores that sell these spoons in gold and platinum for their wealthy clients. In a recent study of drug use among patients between the ages of fifteen and twenty-five who were hospitalized for a "drug problem," the lowest category of use was cocaine among ten classes of drugs. This probably reflects several things: the cost factor, the preference, and the less likely chance of encountering the problems generated by the other classes of drugs.

The issue of use versus abuse is nowhere more clearly defined than in cocaine versus coca leaf chewing. Injected, toxic doses of cocaine at 20 micrograms, and 1.2 grams is fatal. Gilman and Goodman state in their book on the pharmacological basis of therapeutics, "acute poisoning from cocaine is not rare." Further, ill effects are a psychic habituation (not a demonstrable physiological addiction), and depression that follows the effects of the cocaine "high" that is during its duration of activity pleasurable and euphoric. If cocaine is injected, the site of injection is apt to form abscesses due to the vasoconstriction in the area and cocaine acting as a local protoplasmic poison. This is a far cry from the quids of coca leaves that are stashed between the gums and molars in Peru for the slow extraction of cocaine. Among these people, the daily use of coca has had no demonstrable ill effects. These people lead long lives in a society that has had this drug for thousands of years and yet maintained a social structure that has not deteriorated. The recent introduction of distilled alcohol promises to put an end to this, however. There is no medical literature that documents any dangerous effects from chewing coca leaves that are in excess of those associated with normal consumption of coffee or tea.

During the years 1844–1913 Angelo Mariani distributed his wine laced with cocaine to every significant figure in the world and requested a statement and permission to reproduce an image in the *Mariani Albums* consisting of thirteen thick, bound volumes. If the use of this cocainized wine was so pernicious, we would have lost every major head of state, two popes, every significant actress and playwright, composers, etc. The founder of the London Hospital for Throat Diseases considered Vin Mariani a valuable stimulant and stated that he had used the product for many years. The secretary to President William McKinley wrote to Mariani on behalf of the president thanking him for the beverage. We have no indication as to whether McKinley availed himself of the beverage.

In summation, cocaine is a non-addicting stimulant that in large doses may be lethal, but taken in small amounts as leaf material over long time periods would seem to have no significant debilitating effects. Those who classify cocaine with opiates such as heroin and morphine have a profound misunderstanding of the true nature of this stimulant from the Andes.

In an Arabic manuscript of 1333, we find reference to a "tea" made from buds, twigs, and fresh leaves of a woody perennial, *Catha edulis* (Fig. 83). *Khat (quat, chat, tschat, tchai)* is one of several popular names for this brew which predates coffee in Arabia by over one hundred years. Native to northeastern Africa, khat was introduced into the Yemen when the country was dominated by Abyssinia before the sixth century, and it has since found favor throughout much of Africa.

An initial feeling of excitation and gaiety follows consumption of khat, after which a mildly hallucinogenic effect may be experienced. Like coca, it allows an individual to go without food for extended periods of time. Euphoriants to be found in khat include dexedrine, ephedrine, d-norpseudoephedrine, and pervitin. Norpseudoephedrine is the alkaloid predominant in the desert shrub *Ephedra* which was so

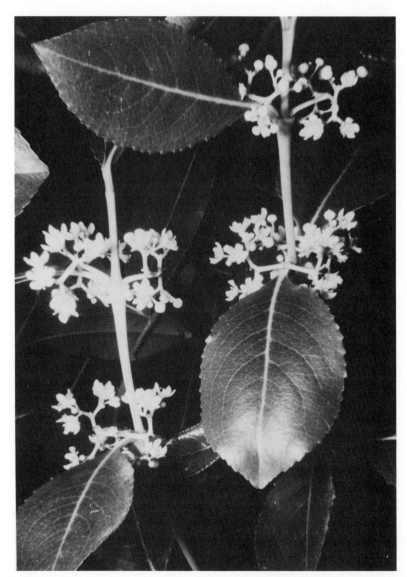

FIG. 83:
Catha edulis

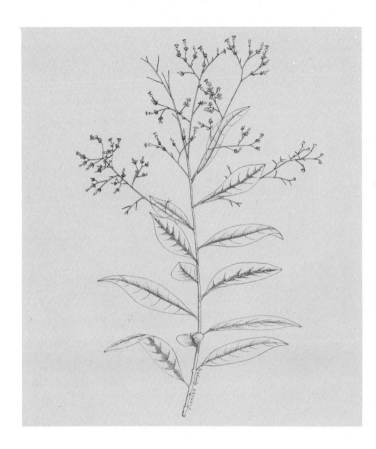

F<small>IG</small>. 84:
Duboisia myoporoides

popular with the early Mormons as the basis for a tea (see Pl. 23). Adverse symptoms often follow a prolonged consumption of khat, for the overstimulation of the heart results in various cardiac diseases. In Yemen, where khat enjoys its greatest popularity, it has been asserted that there are great numbers of bachelors, for the drug presumably reduces sexual drive. Drinking and chewing khat is a social pastime as important to many Africans as the Western coffee break. Yemen and Aden tribes, who have warred for centuries, retire every evening for their khat ritual. So important is khat as a commodity, that its daily export to Aden lies behind the founding of the Ethiopian Airlines.

In the desolate interior of Australia, lack of water and food limits the population of semi-nomadic, aborigine tribes who have learned to live under conditions of great hardship. These people travel trails centuries old that meander through scrub vegetation in the interior of the continent. Commonly called *"pituri* roads,"* they were named after the narcotic shrub in search of which the roads were blazed hundreds of years previous. Leaves of the *pituri (Duboisia hopwoodii* and a taller species, *D. myoporoides)* when roasted, moistened, and rolled into a "quid" have the capacity to ward off hunger, pain, and fatigue—elements common to these tribes living under duress (Fig. 84). It is supposed that numerous alkaloids are

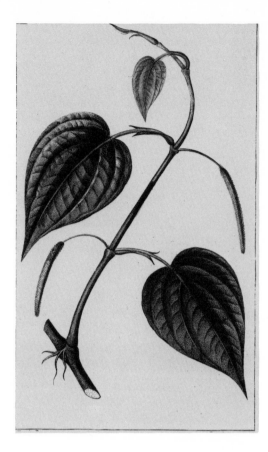

FIG. 85: *Piper betel*

common in these leaves, but the prominent one in *D. myoporoides* is scopolamine, an alkaloid that, even in therapeutic doses, causes excitement and hallucinations. In larger doses it may become fatal. Game animals are captured by the natives by *pituri* poisoning of waterholes where the animals regularly drink.

Pituri is an item of common barter among tribes not living in areas where the plant grows; it is known to these people under twenty different names. Not only do they chew the sausage-like quid, and then swallow the residue, but since the introduction of Europeans to Australia, *pituri* has also been smoked. Although the poisoned dreams of *pituri* represent a flirtation with death, they are preferred to the sting of a harsh reality. Perhaps it is *pituri* that has permitted these people to survive the rigors of this harsh environment for so long.

One of the most popular stimulants since ancient times has been the seed of a palm, *Areca catechu*, which goes under the popular name betel (Pl. 53). To the peoples of southern Asia and the islands of the Indian and Pacific oceans, betel is as important as tobacco is to our culture. A bit of leaf from the vine *Piper betel* (Fig. 85) and a piece of lime are usually mixed with the slice of *Areca* (Fig. 86). Asiatic cultures vary the ingredients to include cloves, tamarind, turmeric, cardamom, and resins. Arecoline is the alkaloid that may act as a very mild stimulant and powerful masticatory (the chewing is accompanied by regular squirts of red saliva). Although the spitting is a menace to health, the arecoline swallowed helps rid these people of some internal parasites.

Betel palms produce about two hundred and fifty seeds or nuts per year, and millions of these trees are under cultivation. Frequent use of betel results in accretion of a lime and pigment residue that blackens teeth. Black teeth are such a mark of distinction that in some island cultures they raise one to the highest social stratum. Because of its astringent properties, betel will probably never enjoy any popularity outside its present distribution, where it is carried in elaborate repositories.

Numerous other stimulants are used by people of the world for similar reasons. Societies deficient in food resort to narcotics that will alleviate the pangs of hunger and concomitant fatigue; where food is plentiful, the fatigue which is the result of boredom or disenchantment is mitigated by similar antidotes.

In all cultures, the quest for altered states of consciousness continues to persist, as it has since the emergence of civilization. Perhaps it is a distinguishing characteristic of civilization that man wishes to govern his states of consciousness as strongly as he desires to govern his physical powers, if only to spend a few moments "lingering in the beautiful foolishness of things."

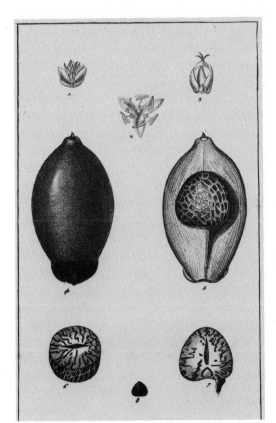

FIG. 86: *Areca catechu*—betelnuts

INEBRIANTS

"I drink Wine not for Pleasure, nor for Profligacy,
nor to renege Religion and good Morals:
but solely to escape a Moment from myself."

The Rubáiyát of Umar Khayyám–*Quatrain 63*
Translated from the French of
J. B. Nicholas by Frederick Baron Corvo

OUT OF ANCIENT PERSIA comes a wondrous legend of a prince who owned a vineyard that provided table grapes and grape juice, which he stored for a time in the skin of sheep. One year when the harvest was particularly bountiful, the prince was able to put aside numerous skins of this delicious juice, which he hoped to consume during the period between harvests. After several weeks he found that much of the juice had become sour, so he had these skins labeled as poison. This same prince had a wife who could not satisfy him in love, and so despondent was the lady that coming upon these skins labeled poison, she consumed cup upon cup of the brew to put an end to her wretched life. To her amazement, the result was not a visitation by the angel of death, but a wonderful sense of joy and buoyancy. She rushed to her husband to reveal this mysterious event and her gaiety and charm left them both fulfilled. From that time forward the brew was celebrated throughout the land as a font of happiness.

Where true origins must remain a mystery, a legend is perhaps the best beginning, and this story from Persia is among the numerous colorful myths explaining the origins of alcohol among the civilizations of man.

Although the world of Islam lays claim to being the origin of enology and viticulture, it is assuredly a derived tradition. The citizens of both Accad and Erech possessed vines and knowledge of wine making. This practice certainly originated in the hills farther north of these cities, but the Sumerians were the first to record their knowledge of the craft. Whether the beginners are to be placed at a date six thousand years ago or eight thousand years ago makes little difference except to ethnobotanists. That which is of considerable importance, however, is the symbolic tradition associated with the spread of wine and viticulture. It is to be expected that a beverage resembling blood and having the power to alter man's conscious state would in any civilization be accorded sacramental usage and might even become considered a substance to be venerated.

In the first epic work ever set down by the hand of man, *The Legend of*

Gilgamesh, deriving from a Sumerian text on clay tablets, the protagonist sets out on a quest for eternal life and almost finds it in a vineyard. When Gilgamesh meets the deity Ishtar, keeper of the sacred vineyard, we are told that the beauty of the grapes is comparable to lapis lazuli (also indicating that it was a blue or purple grape that was then in cultivation), and that the fruit of the vine can impart eternal life. This sacred tradition prevails to this day and has reappeared in major civilizations of the West and Middle East in various guises. Although Gilgamesh is not granted eternal life from the vine, he does find a plant in the bottom of the sea that is capable of the same power; unfortunately, it is stolen by a serpent. The choice of the serpent in this context would not be significant if it did not reappear in subsequent legends.

The Egyptians personified the divine vine in the form of their favorite god, Osiris, brother and husband of Isis. It is said that the body of Osiris was washed up on the shores of Byblos, a cultural center outside of Egypt proper, where it was embalmed. This recapitulates the legends of Ama-Gestin (mother vine-stock) of the Sumerians. Ama-Gestin was the female deity who presided over wine and viticulture. As the tradition moved south into the Nile Delta, the legend changed in two significant ways: Ama-Gestin became Ana-Gestin and instead of presiding over wine, she became patroness of the waters, a process contemporaneous with the migration of the vine and viticulture to the south around 3500 B.C. Secondly, Osiris was the first male figure to preside as god of the vine. Formerly priestesses were enologists, and the lore surrounding the vine personified it as a female entity. The Egyptians of Byblos, however, believed that the vine should be consecrated to Osiris, god of the dead and the underground world of the spirits, and libations should be poured to this god of the realm of shades. Toasts were drunk to one's ghost during life, and wine was offered as nourishment on the journey to that far world. There is some indication that wine was preferred to beer as a libation, for some of the early tomb inscriptions indicate that for a Pharaoh lions were slain and copious libations of fine wines were made to flow. For a lesser person beer was offered, and the brewer had a lesser status. In one instance it is stated that beer was brewed by the keeper of the donkey stable, certainly a decline from the earlier status of priestesses as brewers.

The Greek Herodotus would have us believe that there was no wine in ancient Egypt; this Hellenic conceit comes from the dislike of the Greeks for beer. Thracian allies to the north indulged in the stuff, but Hellas proper spurned malted beverages. It did not seem to occur to Herodotus that the Egyptians might be enjoying both beverages. A period of decline in wine consumption in Egypt seems to coincide with the decline of the great dynasties. It has often been pointed out that the zenith of most civilizations (excepting those of the East) has paralleled the production or consumption of great wines. We do not know how much of the wine consumed in Egypt was imported from the north. Certainly the area of the Nile Delta did not offer appropriate acreage for truly fine wine grapes. The absence of hills and appropriate temperatures would limit the variety of grapes grown as well as the quality. It seems a safe conjecture that much of the wine was imported from allied or conquered lands. With a diminution in power and prestige, the areas that might supply such wines would disappear. Tyre and Sidon were the ancient maritime cities of

Phoenicia and their flourishing viticulture was the pride of West Syria. Their excellent sea trade made vintage wines a major commodity of their economy. It is likely that the Greeks derived their first vintages from such seaport cities. Even though the area of Greece contained numerous wild species of grapes, it seems that they were only considered suitable to be gathered as fruit for the table except for the juice of certain island species which was used for medicine. Black wine from the island of Cos was supposed to allay headaches when mixed with seawater. It is understandable that the Greeks would be receptive to the fine vintages offered them. Enology had progressed to such a degree that the early heavy syrupy wines made from raisins had evolved into a beverage that was reasonably light and potable. The Greeks had a land that was ideally suited to growing numerous varieties of grapes, and they readily introduced viticulture. In fact, it was to the credit of the Greeks that the vines were introduced elsewhere. In every land visited by the Greeks an attempt was made to establish vineyards. A male deity became god of the vine in Greece: Dionysus, Fifth Ruler of the Universe, presided over the vine in Hellas. It is always easy to recognize him in frescoes or reliefs, for he has as his companions a serpent (who stole eternal life from Gilgamesh) and a jaguar. He bears a staff surmounted by one or more pine cones. The latter is probably an allusion to the Greek habit of stoppering amphoras of wine with pitch from the pine, a practice resulting in those wines known today as rezinos. He is often seen with a mountain in the background. Some scholars have identified this as Vesuvius, but Zeus, the father of Dionysus, dwelt on Mount Nysa, and it was there that Dionysus was "born" into his second epiphany. Frequently the god himself is presented as a cluster of grapes assuming the form of a man-god (Fig. 87).

The two epiphanies of Dionysus are integral to an understanding of the success of viticulture in Hellas. In the first epiphany Persephone is incestuously violated by her father, Zeus, husband of Hera, who comes to her in the form of a serpent. The product of this union, the young Dionysus, must pay for Zeus' indiscretion by being boiled and then burned. One version of the story has it that only his heart was spared. From the ashes of the child scattered on the ground there immediately grew the vine—a sacred manifestation of the god as a plant. In one of several versions of the second epiphany the mortal Semele prays for a physical visitation by Zeus. This being impossible, he makes his "entry" as a bolt of lightning, impregnating the naive girl. This dramatic copulation kills Semele, and Zeus out of pity takes the minuscule product of their union, cuts open his thigh and inserts the embryo, which is secured by the daughter of Aristaeus, and then he retires to Mount Nysa to enact the first male pregnancy in history. After a suitable period, Dionysus emerges triumphant. An amusing story, but of profound import. An interpretation of this epiphany that would serve to explain its importance is that Semele, weak and mortal, had the capacity to give birth to a god—the vine. Since the union between a mortal and immortal god was impossible, however, the survival of such a union could only come about through the aforementioned thigh "graft." Mediterranean areas are susceptible to the vine louse *Phylloxera*. Grafting a delicate scion of *Vitis vinifera* (Pl. 54) onto a strong native stock could overcome the resistance of a non-native vine. and permit it to flourish. If this interpretation is correct, it

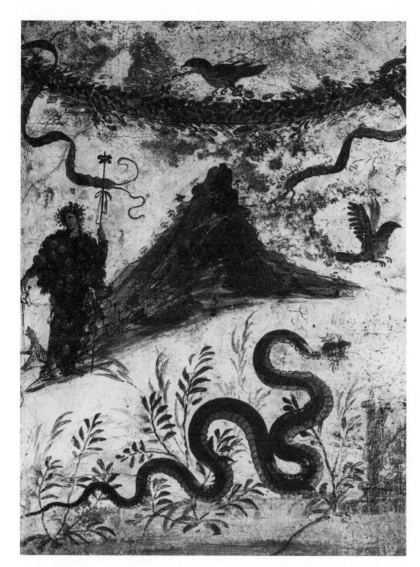

Fig. 87: Dionysus as a
cluster of grapes—
from Pompeii

is the first allusion to grafting of grape vines in history. It may well explain the
success of viticulture in ancient Greece.

    After the conquest of Gaul, the Romans took the lead in the production of fine
wines. The reasons are several: the Roman Empire was spreading into lands suitable
for viticulture; knowledge of storing wines had reached such an art that Petronius
Arbiter could boast of wines over one hundred years old; the vine stocks coming
into Italy represented the finest in the world to date. Lydians sent their vines into
what is now known as Tuscany; Corsica provided a tradition of viticulture, as did
Crete, and vines from both were brought to the mainland; Greek vines were also
welcome. Thus, viticulture among the Romans was a mosaic of independent

traditions that resulted in excellent vintages of every sort. The finest wines paralleled the heyday of the Roman Empire, and the decline was reflected in the deterioration of viticulture and enology. Fortunately, within a hundred years there was a revival in the art of producing wines in these areas, and excellent vintages were being realized.

In Italy the Dionysian tradition was readily assimilated, and the god Bacchus became the Italian version of Dionysus. Also, the act of inebriation began to take on a different color. Whereas Greek writers spoke of the value of wine in keeping a man from a hardened heart, which develops from an overactive intellect, the Romans tended to record, and live, the excesses of Bacchus and his companions the Bacchae. Since Rome in its greatest years consumed twenty-five million gallons of wine per year, excess was the mean. Bacchus is more frequently depicted with his old mentor Silenus in a festive spirit. An early bronze from Pompeii depicts the infant Bacchus held aloft by the spirited Silenus, who bears cymbals and a reed flute. Early Roman writers maintain that an adulterated wine was used at bacchanals in order to induce a frenzied state. Belladonna and henbane have been identified as the primary adulterants of this strong wine, explaining the "hysteria" of the bacchanal, as well as the extended state of somnolence that terminated such rites.

According to Pliny, the vine was the most esteemed plant cultivated by the Romans. A Roman soldier was disciplined by being flogged with a grape vine; a foreigner would be punished by being beaten with any stick at hand. Every major Roman poet celebrated the vine, and even the minor poets could not neglect to sing its praises.

To Islam we owe the fragrant wines made from muscat grapes. Although Koranic injunctions have condemned excesses of intoxication, there is no passage in these sacred writings in which wine is condemned. Indeed, if we look at the history of the origin of the vine it would be Islamic, as it is interpreted in a broad sense. Mount Nysa, birthplace of Dionysus, is said by some to be in Arabia. By the seventh and eighth centuries, Islam produced fine muscat and amber wines. Mahomet's strictures were not a general prohibition, but rather a measure to prevent excesses—especially among the Bedouin soldiers. Such laws are to be interpreted as practical rather than mystical. Overzealous followers of Mahomet ignore such Koranic writings as that in the *Book of the Bee* in which God sends down grapes from which one may obtain an inebriating beverage, "a sign of resurrection unto people who hearken. . . ." That wine was prized among the followers of Mahomet is made clear when in describing eternity it is said that there will be no want of the wine that is prohibited in this life. Early Persian miniatures on goatskin depict wine being consumed by an obviously wealthy household. In one such painting deities are figured among the participants in a "Persian Bacchanal." Wines were not only enjoyed in Islam, but took on a special meaning with respect to decision-making. When the head of a household had to make a decision of importance, he would become intoxicated and offer to members of his house his inebriated deliberations. On the following day his judgement would once more be put before him for consideration. Implicit in such a ritual is the belief that wine intoxication had altered his conscious state in such a way that he might be given over to more profound insights than in sober moments. Does this not compare well with the Greek tradition of not permitting a "hardened heart" to govern life? It is an aspect of divination, or coming to a oneness and prophetic understanding through altering the conscious state. Subliminal judgements would seem to bear degrees of insight not acquired by the rigor of acute conscious intellectualizing.

The Dionysian tradition conquered most of the Western world, but never really succeeded in the East. Before Marco Polo's visits to the East some wine grapes were being grown, but mostly to serve to the Iranians, the only powerful allies that the Chinese had to help fight against the barbaric Turks. On occasions of state the emperor would put a wine on his table, which Marco Polo described as "fragrant and fiery." The fiery nature of the wine has led to speculation by some technologists that the Chinese had come to a method of distillation by freezing that predated that of the Arab world. It is understandable that the Chinese rejected the vine as a major crop, for they had a tradition stressing introspection rather than gregarious Dionysian revelry. Also, as early as the Han dynasty, the Chinese had reached a level of culture that exceeded that of all other nations. Another reason for rejecting wine was that the first introductions were from seed rather than cuttings, and the resultant progeny would be a highly variable mixture of plants that collectively could not produce a high-quality beverage. The most suitable vines, ultimately, were those known as "mares' nipples"—probably a hybrid of *Vitis vinifera* and some native *Vitis* species that bore pale elongated fruits.

Tracing the vine in Western cultures would lead to such parallels as those already described. The consummate civilizations of the West have had their equal in the vintages they produced or imported. Consumption of wine has less connection with its nutritive value than the "feeling of contentment, ease, and comfort that results from imbibing it," to quote from Lewin. The protagonists in the history of wine exemplify its virtues: prophetic Silenus, Dionysus who preserves the wisdom of the heart, and Bacchus who celebrates the joy of living.

Alcohol predates the appearance of man on our planet, for it is the product of certain classes of single-celled organisms splitting sugar molecules into the products of carbon dioxide and alcohol. Fermentation, as this process has been called, occurs whenever sugar and yeast are found together in an aqueous environment. Flowers, fruits, stems, leaves, roots, all plant parts that contain sugar or starches are susceptible to this enzymatic breakdown by living organisms. We have hieroglyphics as well as drawings from ancient Egypt showing the fermentation of grain being carried out to produce alcohol. Among the early Hebrew sects, the fruit of the vine became the most popular source of alcohol, and the practice spread to the Arabs and Coptic Christians, the latter regarding fermentation as an act of the devil. The Bible mentions wine 165 times. In sixteenth-century England we find flowers of the dandelion *(Taraxacum officinale)* being gathered and the nectar fermented to a fine golden-colored wine. At the same time, the Moors were enjoying date wines *(Phoenix dactylifera)*, the Japanese rice wine, the Incas *chicha* from chewed corn *(Zea mays)*, and the Mexicans *Pulque* from the macerated stem and leaf bases of *Agave* species. The Vikings diluted and fermented honey to produce mead which they drank from human skulls with the toast, "skoal." In

Russia the traditional vodka is made from fermented potato tubers *(Solanum tuberosum)*, while in the United States it is produced from wheat. No flower or fruit escapes the scrutiny of man in his quest for inebriants. Even cattle have the sense to feed below apple trees that have dropped their overripe fruit. As the apples ferment, alcohol is produced; few sights are as comical as a herd of drunken cattle.

It is a common assumption that alcohol is a stimulant. This is not the case, for alcohol is a protoplasmic poison acting as a primary and continuous depressant on the central nervous system; furthermore, it is in some instances addictive. It is not the function of this book to deal with alcoholism as a human disease; it is enough to say that great numbers of people in the United States and elsewhere are suffering from alcoholism, a condition that wastes their lives. Taken in moderation, alcohol may serve as a mild euphoriant by suppressing what Freud refers to as the "super-ego." Properly considered a food, alcohol does supply calories as a break-down product of sugar. When used as a substitute for a normal diet, the individual has a real problem. The effect of alcohol as a protoplasmic poison is conspicuous in the production of alcoholic beverages, for when the concentration of alcohol reaches thirteen per cent, it becomes toxic to the organism bringing about fermentation and the process ceases. Thus, concentrations of alcohol above this level are artificially produced. The most serious long-term effect of alcohol on the human body is its interference with normal fat metabolism, especially in the liver where the accumulation of fat causes the organ to become hard and swollen (cirrhosis).

Another of the myths surrounding alcoholic beverages is that they have aphrodisiac properties. Shakespearean jests regarding alcohol are too numerous to quote, but one seems particularly apt. In *Macbeth* (Act II, Sc. III), Macduff asks a porter, "What three things does drink especially provoke?" The porter answers, "Marry, sir, nose-painting, sleep, and urine. Lechery, sir, it provokes and it unprovokes; it provokes the desire, but it takes away the performance: therefore, much drink may be said to be an equivocator with lechery; it makes him and it mars him; it sets him on, and it takes him off; it persuades him and disheartens him; makes him stand to, and not stand to: in conclusion, equivocates him in a sleep, and giving him the lie, leaves him." There is both humor and real understanding of the effects of alcohol in these observations.

In primitive cultures, the making of alcoholic beverages from grain has changed little from the procedures that Columbus observed when, on his third voyage in 1498, he found Indians in the area now known as Venezuela making a crude but tasty beer called *chicha*. Women of the Indian village chew kernels of corn into a pulp, which they spit into a common vessel. Unwittingly, by enzymes in their saliva (salivary amalyases and maltases) they are breaking down the starchy kernels into simpler molecules of sugar that can be acted upon by yeast. Yeast cannot break down starch molecules, and only certain sugars are to its liking. There is no need to add yeast to the pot of mash and spittle, for these microscopic organisms are to be found almost everywhere. For this fungus, a warm, moist container, such as the spittle pot of corn pulp, which has started to change to a sugary brew, is an ideal environment for proliferation. As the fungus reproduces asexually at a considerable rate, it utilizes the sugars to provide energy for its metabolism, giving off ethyl alcohol and carbon dioxide as a byproduct. When the alcohol concentration reaches thirteen per cent, the yeast succumbs to the poison which it has created. No organism can survive if it continues to accumulate poisons in its environment, a lesson man has yet to learn.

While our wines of today are produced with an almost infallible skill that assures a consistent quality never experienced by any past generations, it is estimated that over half of the wine produced by the Egyptians and Romans was spoiled because of exposure to air and organisms that can convert the beverage into vinegar. This was overcome by the Greeks, as mentioned earlier; they learned to stop the bottles with resin or pine pitch, a process that insured against spoilage, but usually flavored the wine to a considerable degree. Greece has, however, developed a taste for resinous wines and, although such procedures are no longer necessary, a bit of pitch is sometimes introduced to flavor the wine.

Another tale surrounding spirit production is that of the Benedictine monk Dom Perignon, cellarer at The Abbey of Hautvilliers, who when assisting in the production of sacramental wine in 1679, stoppered some bottles of wine before fermentation had been completed, thus causing the bubbles of carbon dioxide to accumulate. This fortunate mistake is said to have been the origin of champagne. The best champagne and sparkling burgundy is still produced by a premature sealing of the bottle of fermenting grape juice; poorer substitutes are produced by artificially introducing bubbles of carbon dioxide. The art and science of wine making has reached such levels of complexity that some universities now offer programs leading to degrees in this area. Enology, the study of wine production, is not to be confused with viticulture, the study of producing the grapes; granted, they are complementary disciplines.

Whenever a civilization has had a grain crop, that same culture has produced beer. There is reason to believe that the infant civilization of man was nursed on beer. Mesopotamia has been called by anthropologists "the cradle of civilization," and in the earliest Sumerian and Akkadian writings on clay tablets taken from recent excavations there is reference to "beer" as a part of man's daily wage. Since barley (*Hordeum* sp.) was the grain of this civilization, we may assume that the brew was a fermented product of this cereal.

In Babylonia, the goddess Siris was the patroness of beer (later to be replaced by Ninkasi). Temple priestesses were also women brewers and produced several different kinds of beer; over six classes are mentioned by name. Some of these beers were used as a food and beverage for general consumption, but a few were retained by the priestesses for temple rites. Shu-bad, Queen of Mesopotamia, drank her beer from a golden cup and through a golden straw. Mash byproducts of this ancient brewery were used to fatten cattle and were formed into cakes as a sort of bread.

One of history's most intriguing writings is an Egyptian manuscript known as the Papyrus of Ani which dates c. 4000 B.C. In this tome we find reference to an intoxicant, *hek*, made from grain. The description of the beverage establishes it as beer. *Hemki*, a modification of the word *hek*, has persisted as an Egyptian word until comparatively recent times. Egyptian medical treatises of five thousand years ago list over one hundred medicines that use beer as a base. So esteemed was the brew that it was offered as a libation by Rameses III in the form of thirty thousand gallons annually. By the year 3000 B.C., inebriation had become a problem in this ancient civilization, and repressive measures had to be initiated.

Legends of ancient Egypt ascribe the origin of beer to Osiris, who taught Egypt the art of brewing from barley grain and grapes. We know that beer, like wine, was offered as sustenance for the journey after death, and one of the toasts proposed while drinking beer was "Here's beer for your spirit." Unfortunately, some of the sources recording the use of beer in ancient Egypt are the writings of classical Greek writers such as Aeschylus, who believed that the beer of these early dynasties was so poor that only women could drink it.

In the Bible, the book of Deuteronomy relates an admonition to the Nazarenes to abstain from "strong drink," and in Leviticus priests are forbidden to drink "strong drink" before going to the tabernacle. The Hebrew word *sicera* (strong drink) is thought by some scholars to be barley beer, which the Israelites learned to brew from the Egyptians. It is a Rabbinical tradition that the captive Jews in Babylon remained free from leprosy by drinking *siceram ex lupulis confectam*, or barley beer made bitter with the addition of hops (*Humulus lupulus*, Fig. 88).

Pliny tells us that all the nations of western Europe had an intoxicating beverage of corn and water, and he notes that "so exquisite is the ingenuity of mankind . . . that they have invented a method of making water itself intoxicate." Dioscorides in the first century B.C. records the use of *curmi*, a barley beer, by the Britons. Diodorus Siculus recorded that these Britons drank barley beer only on festive occasions, usually preferring water, and afterwards often became quarrelsome.

The Library of Congress in Washington, D.C., has a journal kept by a passenger on the *Mayflower*. The entry under 19 December 1620 states that a landing of the ship at Plymouth was made because "we could not now take time for further search or consideration: our victuals being much spent, especially our beere. . . ." Eight years before the Pilgrims set foot in North America a brewery flourished on Manhattan Island. In 1637 the Massachusetts Bay Colony gave Captain Robert Sedgwick a license to operate the first brewery in New England. Samuel Adams, signer of the Declaration of Independence, inherited a brewery from his father and became known for the quality of his brew. Likewise, Thomas Jefferson, George Washington, James Madison, and Patrick Henry were all brewers. Jefferson went so far as to send to Bohemia for brewers so that they might teach their art to Americans.

The record of brewing is extensive; however, it is not the chronology that is important, but the fact that it points to the end of man's nomadic existence and the establishment of agricultural practices associated with civilization. It is interesting to note that beer, like wine, has been used not only as a refreshing beverage, but as a sacrificial offering or libation in temples.

Beer production is an industry of considerable importance in California, where some of the world's largest and most elaborate breweries are to be found. Brewing begins with germination of barley seeds, a crop occupying extensive acreage in northern California. Malt represents a partial enzymatic breakdown of the storage

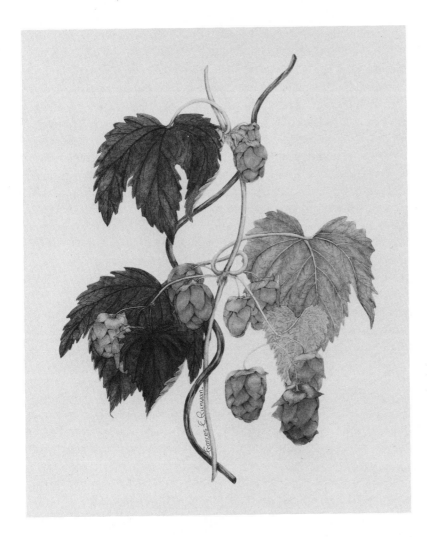

F<small>IG</small>. 88:
Humulus lupulus

products (endosperm) of the grain. After two days of steeping the barley in cold water, the grain is left to sprout for four to six days and then the process is stopped by dry roasting at 180 degrees Fahrenheit (higher if a dark beer is desired). To this malt is added thirty-five per cent of other grains, such as rice, corn, etc., to make a mash which is soaked at temperatures conducive to its further enzymatic break-down (the mixture is then known as wort). Liquid wort is drained off and boiled with hops for several hours to give the bitter flavor that beer drinkers prize. The female inflorescence is used for the complex oils found in glandular hairs on those flowers.

In Rome the hop plant was known as *Lupus salictarius*, or "wolf among wil-lows," for where it grew among the willows, it was as destructive as a wolf among sheep. It was from this tradition that Linnaeus derived the specific epithet *lupulus*. No doubt the use of hops by the Jews during their Babylonian captivity to prevent leprosy indicates the origin of adding hops to beer. Not only were hops considered as being of medicinal value, but Pliny mentions in his *Natural History* that the Germans used hops to preserve their ale. In spite of the preservative powers of hops, it took centuries to condition the English taste to the bitter vine. German hop gardens were fairly common by the eighth century, but hops were not mentioned in brewing until A.D. 1097 when the Abbess Hildegard of Rupertsburg wrote in her *Physica Sacia*, "If one intends to make beer from oats it is prepared with hops."

Bitter wort with hops is taken to starting cellars where strains of yeast (*Saccharomyces cerevisiae*) are introduced to initiate fermentation under cool conditions. Complex procedures follow, but the basic pattern is the further breakdown of sugars to yield alcohol and carbon dioxide, the latter providing a head of foam on the final product. Beer in the market contains about five per cent alcohol, malt, and sugar. Variants of beer are numerous and usually involve the substitution of grains other than barley and a change in the quantity of hops. Sometimes, however, as in the making of *chicha* in South America, numerous plant parts are used, including fruits, so that at certain points, beer and wine become indistinguishable.

We have spoken thus far only of the gentle spirits produced for thousands of years whose alcoholic content does not exceed thirteen per cent. But what of the distiller's craft that has brought us whisky, brandy, gin, vodka, rum, and a host of liqueurs? We know that by the tenth century A.D. the Arabs had stills in which they made use of the principle that alcohol has a lower boiling point than water and may, as a volatile substance, be cooled and trapped as a liquid. Nowadays, distillers in the United States are producing close to eight hundred million gallons of distilled spirits for consumption annually. This compares favorably with the almost three hundred million gallons of wine and two hundred million barrels of beer per annum. Statistics corresponding with these are the five hundred million dollars of wages lost each year because of alcoholism and the estimate that seventy per cent of the homicides in the United States are associated with alcohol consumption by one or both parties. Few people would claim that prohibition accomplished little more than encouraging a criminal black market and the production of "booze" that was often toxic and fatal. Perhaps there is consolation in figures indicating that the per capita consumption of alcohol in the United States has dropped by about forty per cent since 1910. I would attribute this in part to the enormous increase in the use of another "release agent"—*Cannabis*. Dr. Goddard, formerly of the United States Department of Health and Welfare, has stated that marijuana is no more dangerous than alcohol. However, he qualified his statement by citing the social problems created by excesses in alcohol consumption. One major difference is that the physiological addiction that alcohol creates is not to be found in users of marijuana. It is estimated that five per cent of the population of the United States is addicted to alcohol and can be classified as alcoholic. Perhaps the wisdom of St. Paul's counsel to Timothy, "use a little wine for thy stomach's sake and thine own infirmities," is in the qualification, "little."

We cannot escape the conclusion that the origins of inebriating beverages are as many as the origins of human cultures, and like all psychotropic agents, alcohol has provided a respite from the growing pains of infant civilizations and a relief from the burgeoning problems of "mature" mankind. Perhaps one of the most neglected aspects of man is, as Aldous Huxley has pointed out, his desire to transcend himself.

In the words of Housman:

Malt does more than Milton can
to justify God's ways to man.

ALCOHOLIC BEVERAGES FROM PLANTS

Beverage	Primary area of production	Genera of plants	Part used
WINES			
Grape	Europe and US	*Vitis*	fruit
Flower	Europe (England)	*Taraxacum* and *Primula*	flower
Berry	Europe and US	*Prunus, Rubus, Sambucus*	fruit
Mead	Scandinavia and Africa	numerous	honey from flowers
BEERS			
Ale	Germany and US	*Saccharomyces, Humulus,* and *Hordeum*	barley grain
Kvass (Quass)	Russia	*Hordeum, Secale, Mentha*	grains (barley, rye) or rye bread plus peppermint leaves
Pombe (Bousa)	Africa	*Eleusine*	millet grain
Porter	Germany and England	*Hordeum* and *Humulus*	barley grain, malted and carmelized

Beverage	Primary area of production	Genera of plants	Part used
Stout	Germany and England	*Hordeum* and *Humulus*	barley and many hops
Weiss	Germany	*Triticum* and *Humulus*	wheat grain and hops
Chicha	South America	primarily *Zea* and *Chenopodium*	grains of corn or *quinca*
Cider	England and US (North)	*Malus (Pyrus)*	apple
Ginger Beer	England	*Zingiber*	rhizome oils and beer
Palm Toddy	Africa and the Orient	several spp. of palm	sap from wounded inflorescence
Pulque	Mexico	*Agave*	fermented leaf bases
Sake	Japan	*Oriza* fermented by *Aspergillus* fungus	steamed rice, hydrolized and fermented
Sorgho	Africa and Asia	*Sorghum*	grain

DISTILLED SPIRITS

Brandy	Europe and US	*Vitis* primarily	Fruit wine, distilled and aged in wood
Whiskies	Scotland and US	*Zea* and *Secale*	Corn and rye grain malted, fermented, distilled and aged in white oak (charred) casks

Beverage	Primary area of production	Genera of plants	Part used
Gin	England and US	*Zea, Secale,* and *Juniperus*	Corn and rye grains, malted and fermented. To the distillate juniper berries (cones) are added
Rum	Jamaica	*Saccharum*	Distilled, fermented sugar; cane juice carmelized
Absinth	France	*Vitis* and *Artemesia*	Brandy and a narcotic worm-wood
Akvavit	Scandinavia	*Solanum tuberosum, Carum*	Potato dis-tillate with caraway seed for flavor
Oke	Hawaii	*Oriza, Saccharum*	Molasses, rice distillate fer-mented in charred barrels
Tequila	Mexico	*Agave*	Leaf base and stem tissue of *Agave* fer-mented and distilled
Vodka	Russia	*Solanum tuberosum* or *Triticum*	Distillate of potato tubers, or wheat malt

APPENDIX I

A Proposed Structuring of Some Known Mind-Altering Plant Chemicals

The psychopharmacology of mind-altering plants is so complex that a single plant may have multiphasic effects due to its chemistry or according to dosage. A single drug may have an action syndrome ranging from an initial state of light-headedness through a period of fascination, then into a period of bizarre visions that terminates in somnolence.

Although limited to Mexican sacred plants, the classification of José Luis Diaz in 1977 is perhaps the best model to date upon which one might build a systematic classification for the entire world of psychotropic plants. The following is based upon the proposals of Diaz with modification to include representatives from throughout the world. Diaz defines "psychodysleptic" as a plant that is capable of producing "varying degrees of affective, perceptual, imaginative, and thought modifications," and he establishes families of psychodysleptics by their similar subjective effects, cross-tolerance and structure-activity relationships. Psycho-analeptics, on the other hand, produce exhilaration, mental and physical stimulation, and a feeling of well-being.

PSYCHODYSLEPTICS

VISIONARY PSYCHODYSLEPTICS: These plants produce perceptual distortion, a wide range of changing emotional states, distinct and disjunct changes in memory and the thought processes, dissociative reactions, visions, and ecstasy. In some individuals depression, panic, and depersonalization may be manifested.

PHENETHYLAMINES produce euphoria, exhilaration, and sometimes visions. The neuropsychopharmacology of most is poorly understood.

Cactaceae

Lophophora diffusa	*Trichocereus pachanoi*
Lophophora williamsii	*Trichocereus terschekii*
Pelecyphora aselliformis	*Trichocereus werdermannianus*
Trichocereus macrogonus	

INDOLES constitute the nuclear structure of several classes of hallucinogens.

Apocynaceae

Catharanthus lanceus	*Tabernanthe iboga*
Catharanthus roseus	

TRYPTAMINES

Acanthaceae

Justicia pectoralis var. *stenophylla*

Agaricaceae

Conocybe cyanopus
Conocybe siligineoides
Paneolus foenisecii
Paneolus sphinctrinus
Psilocybe acutissima
Psilocybe albida
Psilocybe ambrophila
Psilocybe aztecorum
Psilocybe baeocystis
Psilocybe caerulescens
Psilocybe caerulipes
Psilocybe cordispora
Psilocybe cubensis
Psilocybe cyanescens
Psilocybe fagicola
Psilocybe hoogshagenii
Psilocybe isauri
Psilocybe kumaneorum
Psilocybe mazatecorum
Psilocybe mexicana
Psilocybe mixaeensis
Psilocybe muliercula
Psilocybe nigripes
Psilocybe pelliculosa
Psilocybe semilanceata
Psilocybe semperviva
Psilocybe wassonii
Psilocybe yungensis
Psilocybe zapotecorum

Malpighiaceae

Banisteriopsis caapi
Banisteriopsis inebrians
Banisteriopsis quitensis
Banisteriopsis rusbyana

Mimosaceae

Anadenanthera peregrina
Mimosa hostilis
Mimosa verrucosa

Myristicaceae

Virola calophylla
Virola calophylloidea
Virola rufula
Virola sebifera
Virola theiodora

Rubiaceae

Psychotria viridis

ISOAXZOLES

Agaricaceae

Amanita muscaria

BETA-CARBOLINES

Malpighiaceae

Banisteriopsis caapi
Banisteriopsis inebrians
Banisteriopsis parensis

Zygophyllaceae

Peganum harmala

IMAGERY-INDUCING PSYCHODYSLEPTICS: This group characteristically produces visual imagery, sensations of body-weight changes, memory alterations, time-perception changes, fragmented thinking, and less often delusions.

COUMARINS (may be modified to benzopyrans)

Asteraceae

Artemisia absinthium   *Tagetes lucida*
Calea zacatechichi

DIBENZYOPYRANS

Cannabaceae

Cannabis indica   *Cannabis ruderalis*
Cannabis sativa

PHENYLPROPENES

Myristicaceae

Myristica fragrans

POLYHYDRIC ALCOHOLS

Lamiaceae

Lagochilus inebrians

TRANCE-INDUCING PSYCHODYSLEPTICS: These compounds resemble those in the previous category but have strong characteristics of provoking mental apathy, quietude, lethargy, serenity, and abstract thought.

ERGOLINES

Convovulaceae

Argyreia nervosa   *Rivea corymbosa*
Ipomoea violaceae and *I. carnea*   *Stictocardia* species

Hypocreaceae

Claviceps glabra   *Claviceps paspali*
Claviceps nigricans   *Claviceps purpurea* (fungus - Ascomycete)

OPIATES: Codeine, morphine, thebaine

Papaveraceae

Escholzia california   *Papaver somniferum*

DELIRIANT PSYCHODYSLEPTICS: Chemicals in this category are known to promote confused thinking and subsequent speech disorders. Clouded consciousness and anxiety accompany hallucinations.

TROPANES

Solanaceae

Datura species   *Mandragora officinarum*
Hyoscyamus niger   *Methysticodendron amesianum*
Latua pubiflora

NEUROTOXIC PSYCHODYSLEPTICS: These neural toxins produce profound effects upon peripheral nerual functions and motor coordination. These are in addition to the psychological effects that may mimic trance states and the delirium provoked by the previous categories. Vomiting and a state of stupor are common.

QUINOLIZIDINES

Fabaceae

Cytisus canariensis   *Sophora secundaflora*

Lythraceae

Heimia salicifolia

ERYTHRINANES

Fabaceae

Erythrina species

PYRROLIZIDINES

Asteraceae

Senecio species

PSYCHOANALEPTICS

Psychoanaleptics differ from all aforementioned categories in that they provoke physical and mental stimulation, enhance thought processes, and give one a general sense of clarity and well-being.

COCAINE

Erythroxylaceae

Erythroxylum coca

EPHEDRINE

Celastraceae

Catha edulis

Gnetaceae

Ephredra species (56 in all)

XANTHINES

Aquifoliaceae

Ilex paraguayensis

Malvaceae

Sida acuta

Rubiaceae

Coffea arabica

Sapindaceae

Paullinia cupana

Sterculiaceae

Cola nitida   *Theobroma cacao*

Theaceae

Thea sinensis

Turneraceae

Turnera diffusa

APPENDIX II

A Summation of the Botany Geography, Psychopharmacology and Chemistry of Narcotic Plants

This appendix is an abbreviated synopsis of those plants figured in the text. Where several different species of a genus are mentioned, a characteristic species has been chosen to represent the narcotic members of that genus. Common names have been chosen either because they are commonly used in the area to which the plant is indigenous or are widely used. Species names, as well as generic names, correspond to those in current use. Where a name is abundant in the literature, although a synonym, it is presented as well in parentheses following the most frequently used citation. Authors of the species appear in this appendix but not in the text. These will be found immediately following the specific epithet. The narcosis corresponds to the traditional categories represented in the text rather than the categories that have been proposed in Appendix I. The author is aware that such simplification of a behavioral syndrome is imperfect, and the reader is referred to the text and Appendix I for a more complete characterization of the narcosis.

Entries are alphabetized according to genus and species. Question marks have been introduced where the narcosis is based upon inconclusive reports or where the nature of the active principle is in doubt or has not been established with certainty.

The following arrangement is used throughout this appendix:
Genus species (both in italics) Author (s)   Local or common name
Family
Habitat
Botanical description
Primary narcotic effect
Active principle(s)

Acorus calamuus L.   "Sweet Flag," "Sweet Calomel"
Araceae
Northern United States and Canada
In bogs or marshy areas
Terrestrial herb from creeping rootstock; leaves sword-shaped, to 25 cm or more; the lateral greenish spadix, 5–16 cm long, spathe narrow and not prominent.
Mild hallucinogen
Beta-asarone

Actaea alba (L.) (Mill. *A. pachypoda* Ell.)   "White Baneberry"
Ranunculaceae
Eastern Canada south to Georgia, Louisiana, and Oklahoma
Rich wooded areas
Perennial herb, to 1 m tall; leaves large, 2–3 ternately compound; leaflets sharply toothed; flowers small, white in a dense long-peduncled terminal raceme; berries white, with a persistent stigma.
Hypnotic
Unidentified

Actinidia polygama (Sieb. & Zucc.) Maxim.   "Chinese Cat Powder"
Actinidiaceae
Japan
Thickets and woods in mountains
A deciduous, scandent shrub; leaves ovate to elliptic 6–15 cm long; often leaves near the inflorescence white on upper half of upper side; flowers axillary, white, pendulous with many stamens; fruit a berry.
Tranquilizer with mild hallucinogenic effects
Metatabilacetone and actinidine

Aesculus glabra Willd.   "Ohio Buckeye"
Hippocastanaceae
Central and Eastern United States but not along the southeast coast
Woods, thickets, base of bluffs
Tree to 17 m tall; leaves palmately compound with 5–7 leaflets; flowers greenish-yellow in many flowered, large panicles; fruit prickly with shiny, large, dark-brown seeds.
Hypnotic
Aesculin (esculin)

Aesculus pavia L.   "Red Buckeye"
Hippocastanaceae
Most of the Eastern United States
Moist deciduous forests, low woodlands and swamp margins
Shrub or small tree to 4 m tall; leaves palmately compound with leaflets up to 8 cm long; flowers scarlet in a terminal panicle; capsule to 7 cm in diameter with light-brown seeds.
Hypnotic
Aesculin (esculin)

Alchornea floribunda Müll. Arg.   "Niando"
Euphorbiaceae
West Tropical Africa, Congo, Uganda
Forests
A leaning, semi-climbing shrub or small tree to 10 m; leaves obovate-oblanceolate, 20–35 cm long; flowers dioecious, in branched inflorescences, green; fruits capsular.
Hallucinogen
Yohimbine (questionable)

Amanita muscaria L.   "Fly Agaric"
Agaricaceae
Temperate areas throughout the world
Under birch, pine beech, and larch trees in forests
Gilled mushroom appearing quite red-orange in the button stage and maturing into fungus
    8–10 cm in height with an equally broad cap turning tan with white flecks on the hymen
    at maturity.
Hallucinogen
Ibotenic acid and muscimole

Anadenanthera colubrina (Vell.) Brenan   "Vilca," "Cebil"
Mimosaceae
Peru, Bolivia, Argentina
Forests
A tree, often attaining a height of 30 m; leaves compound, 12–20 cm long, pinna pairs, 7–35,
    leaflets, 20–80 pairs; flower heads globose, white to yellow to orange; pods 10–32 cm
    long, 8–16 seeded.
Hallucinogen
N, N-dimethyltryptamine, and related tryptamines

Anadenanthera peregrina Speg.   (*Piptadenia peregrina* Benth.)
                                       "Yopa," "Cohoba," "Parica"

Colombia, Venezuela, Brazil
Forests
A shrub or tall tree, 3–27 m; leaves compound, 10–20 cm long, pinna pairs 10–30 or more,
    leaflets, 25–80 pairs; flower heads globose, axillary, greenish white to yellowish; pods
    5–30 cm long, 8–16 seeded.
Hallucinogen
N, N-dimethyltryptamine, and related tryptamines

Arctostaphylos uva-ursi L.   "Bear-berry," "Kinnikinnick"
Ericaceae
Circumpolar, with its varieties
On sandy or rocky soil
Prostrate shrub forming mats to 1 m across; leaves evergreen, leathery, oblanceolate to
    oblong-obovate, 1–2 cm long; flowers urn-shaped, whitish fruits, round, bright red and
    mealy inside.
Hypnotic
Arbutin and ericolin (these do not explain the narcotic effects)

Areca catechu L.   "Betel Nut," "Areca Nut"
Palmae
India, Malaya, Polynesia
Ubiquitous on South Pacific Islands
A slender tree to 25 m; trunk ringed; leaf blades to 1 m across with many pinnae;
    inflorescence conspicuous, much-branched; fruit ovoid, orange-scarlet, to 5 cm long.
Slight stimulant
Arecoline

Argemone mexicana L.   "Prickly Poppy"
Papaveraceae
Southwestern United States, Mexico
Dry soil in fields and along roadsides
Coarse, prickly, herbaceous perennial with yellow sap; leaves spiny, 10–15 cm long; flowers
    bright yellow, many stamens; fruit a prickly capsule.
Questionable hallucinogen
Imperfectly known

Argyreia nervosa (Burm.) Bojer. "Silver Morning-glory," "Hawaiian Baby Wood Rose"
Convolvulaceae
Tropical Asia; pantropic in cultivation; used in Hawaii
Semi-forested areas: vine
A coarse silvery liana with cordate leaves to 12 cm long and almost as broad; branches,
    undersides of leaves and outer surface of corolla covered with silvery-white hairs; corolla
    funnelform, pale-violet-pink within; fruit a capsule with persistent spreading sepals.
Hallucinations
Ergolines (amides of lysergic acid)

Artemisia absinthium L.   "Wormwood," "Absinth"
Asteraceae
Most of Europe, except the islands
Rocks, screes, uncultivated ground
Much-branched, aromatic, silvery perennial with finely divided leaves with silky hairs on
    both sides; flowers borne in lateral clusters to form a branched pyramidal inflorescence.

Hypnotic; dream delirium
Coumarins, absinthin, absinthol

Atropa belladonna L.   "Deadly Nightshade," "Belladonna"
Solanaceae
Central and southern Europe, southwest Asia, Algeria
Wooded hills in shaded areas
A suffrutescent, perennial herb, to 1.5 m tall; leaves ovate, paired, one leaf of each pair larger
    than the other, 6–18 cm long; flowers bell-shaped, pendant, dingy purple tinged with
    green; fruit a many-seeded shiny black berry
Hallucinogen
Atropine and scopolamine

Banisteriopsis caapi Morton   "Ayahuasca," "Caapi," "Yajé," "Natem pinde"
Malpighiaceae
Brazil, Colombia, Ecuador, Peru
Rain forest

A liana with lenticellate bark; leaves ovate to lanceolate, about 17 cm long, 609 cm wide; flowers in axillary panicles, carmine-pink, petals quick falling; fruit a reddish-brown samara.

Hallucinogen

Harmine, harmaline, d-tetrahydroharmine (tryptamines in *B. rusybana*)

Boletus (Tubiporus) Reayi Heim   "Nonda ngam-ngam"

Polyporaceae

New Guinea (Wahgi Valley)

Forest (especially growing under *Castanopsis acuminatissima*)

A fleshy fungus with a spongy or porous underside to the cap; the tubular stratum peeling from the upper portion of the cap with some ease; cap from 8–25 cm broad and stipe 2–4 cm thick.

Hallucinogen (?)

Unidentified

Brunfelsia tastevini Benoist   "Keya-honé"

Solanaceae

Brazil

Rain forest

A scandent shrub, sometimes a liana; leaves lanceolate, 6–15 cm long; flowers in terminal cymes; corolla tubular, yellowish-white; fruit a berry.

Hallucinogen

Imperfectly known; possibly tropanes, coumarins and the alkaloid scopoletin

Calliandra anomala (Kunth) Macbride   "Cabeza de Angel"

Mimosaceae

Mexico and Guatemala

In level or mountainous places and sometimes along streams

A shrub, 1–4.5 m high; bark blackish, leaves compound with numerous leaflets, 2.5–5 mm long; flowers showy, purple-red, the stamens long-exserted; pod densely hirsute.

Hypnotic

Unidentified principle found in the resins

Calea zacatechichi Schlecht.   "Thle pela kano"

Asteraceae

Mexico and Guatemala

Level places or hillsides

A multi-branched shrub, to 1 m tall; leaves broadly ovate-triangular, 2–6 cm long; flowers in dense cymose-umbellate panicles, rays white; fruit an achene, 1 mm long.

Hallucinogen (primarily visual)

Unidentified coumarins and lactones

Canavalia maritima (Aubl. Thouars)   "Bay Bean," "Frijol de Mar"
Fabaceae
Pantropical shore plant
Beaches and seaside dunes
Trailing vine; leaves trifoliolate, obovate to suborbicular; flowers racemous, rosy-purple; fruit a legume prominently ribbed on each side of the upper suture.
Euphoriant similar to *Cannabis*
1-Betonicine

Cannabis indica Lam.   "Bhang," "Hashish," "Ganja," "Hasheesh"
Cannabaceae
India, Pakistan, Iran, etc. (cultivated in many areas)
Waste places, cultivated in many areas
Densely branched shrub, rarely exceeding 3 m; leaves palmate, alternate; stems rounded (short fibers in phloem); seeds small, globose, heavily marbled. Alternate branching.
Mild euphoria to vivid hallucinations
Delta-1-tetrahydrocannabinol and isomers

Cannabis ruderalis Jan.   "Weedy Hemp"
Cannabaceae
Southeast Russia
Cultivated fields
Unbranched shrub; not exceeding 1.5 m in height; similar to *C. sativa* but differing in its smaller size, its achene with a marbled surface, distinctly articulated at the base and easily detached.
Mild euphoria or no effects
Delta-1-tetrahydrocannabinol

Cannabis sativa L.   "Hemp," "Pot," "Grass," "Marihuana," etc.
Cannabaceae
India, cosmopolitan
Waysides, disturbed places
A coarse, strong-smelling, glandular erect annual or perennial, to 14 m tall; leaves palmate with 3–9 lance-shaped, toothed segments; flowers dioecious, the staminate in long-panicled racemes, pistillate in short leafy axillary glomerules; fruit an achene. Opposite branching.
Mild euphoriant
Delta-1-tetrahydrocannabinol

Casimiroa edulis La. Lla. v.   "Zapote Blanco," "Cochiztzapotl"
Rutaceae
Mexico
Mountain forests; often cultivated

Large tree with a broad dense crown; leaflets 5, elliptic to broadly ovate; flowers small, greenish white; fruit a globose drupe, yellowish with sweet pulp.
Sedating hypnotic
N-benzoyltyramine, methylhistamine, casimiroin, fagarine, and casimirodine

Catha edulis (Vahl) Forsk.   "Khat"
Celastraceae
Arabia
Forest or woodland
A shrub or tree, 2–15 m tall; leaves oblong to elliptic, 5.5–11 cm long; flowers in axillary cymes, small, greenish-yellow; fruit capsular with 1–3 seeds.
Stimulant leading to hallucinations; terminating in somnolence
Ephedrine

Catharanthus roseus Don.   "Madagascar Periwinkle"
Apocynaceae
Originating in Madagascar, now cosmopolitan; used in United States
Grows in a wide variety of soils, exposures, and climate
Erect everblooming herb or subshrub, 12–25 cm high; leaves oblong, 2–6 cm long; flowers white, rosy-purple or lavender with reddish eye, to 3 cm across; corolla tube narrow, 2 cm long.
Hallucinogen (highly toxic)
Ibogaine-like alkaloids

Cimicifuga racemosa L.   "Black Cohosh"
Ranunculaceae
Much of the Eastern USA
Moist or dry woods
Tall perennial herb, 1–2 m high, with large, ternately and pinnately decompound leaves; leaflets coarsely and sharply toothed; inflorescence, a many-flowered, simple, or branched raceme; flowers small, petals lacking; fruit a follicle with roughened seeds.
Hypnotic
Cimicifugin (imperfectly characterized)

Cineraria aspera Thunb.   "Mohodu-wa-pela"
Asteraceae
South Africa
Sunny, well-drained slopes
A suffrutescent perennial 0.5 m or more tall; stems, leaves and flowers heads white woolly-floccose; leaves runcinate-pinnatified, 4–8 cm long; flower heads yellow.
Hallucinogen of questionable status
Unknown

Claviceps purpurea (Fries) Tulasne   "Ergot"
Hypocreaceae
North temperate regions of the world
Parasite of rye flowers
Infected rye flowers produce a sclerotium of mycelium supplanting the ovary turning dark
    purple.
Hallucinogen
Ergine, ergonovine, ergotamine, etc. (numerous alkaloids)

Coffea arabica L.   "Arabian Coffee"
Rubiaceae
Arabia, Tropical Africa
Shrub areas on hillsides
A shrub or a small tree, 3–5 m tall; leaves elliptic, 6–12 cm long, glossy; flowers white, in
    axillary clusters; fruit a 2-seeded deep crimson berry.
Stimulant
Caffeine

Cola nitida (Vent.) Schott. & Endl.   "Cola Nut"
Sterculiaceae
Senegal to Nigeria, Sierra Leone, Ghana, Ivory Coast
Forest
A tree, 10–25 m tall; leaves variable, often obovate, 12–16 cm long; flowers whitish or
    pale-yellow with dark red stripes; fruits of 5 recurved follicles with as many as 10 seeds
    in 2 rows.
Stimulant
Caffeine

Coleus blumei Benth.   "El Macho," "El Nene," "El Ahijado"
Labiatae
Southeast Asia (cultivated in Mexico)
Damp shady places
A perennial herb or sub-shrub, to 1 m tall; leaves toothed, ovate, variously colored, 4–8 cm
    long; flowers blue, in branched racemes; corolla to 12 mm long; fruit a nutlet.
Hallucinogen (?)
Unidentified

Conocybe sp.   "Magic Mushroom"
Agaricaceae
Narcotic sp. Mexico
Fields, gardens, bare soil, mosses, greenhouses, decayed wood, charcoal, anthills, dung, etc.
Pileus hygrophanous, glistening when dry; veil none; spores deep, rich rust color; stipe
    straight and central, elongate and thin, rarely thick or fleshy, often villous or pubescent;
    lamellae usually at first strongly adscendate.
Hallucinogen
Psilocybin

Coriaria thymifolia Humb. & Bonpl.   "Shanshi"
Coriariaceae
Ecuadorian Andes
Mostly on steep cliffs or terraces
A slender shrub, 1–3 m tall, with distichous leaves on short lateral branches, all spreading in
  one plane, 1–2 cm long; flowers tiny in slender racemes; fruits dark-purple, 3–4 mm in
  diameter, juicy.
Hallucinogen giving a sensation of flight
Sesquiterpenes: coriamyrtine, coriatine, tutine, and pseudotutine

Cypripedium calceolus L. var. *pubescens* Willd. (Correll) "Yellow Ladyslipper"
Orchidaceae
Northeastern Canada, south to Georgia, west to Arizona and New Mexico
Shaded woods
Terrestrial orchid to 20 cm tall; leaves 3–5, somewhat 2-ranked, plicate, sheathing the stem;
  flowers showy, large; inflated lip dull to bright yellow outside, spotted dark red or purple
  on the inside.
Hypnotic, sedation, and lassitude
Unidentified

Cytisus canariensis (L.) (*Genista canariensis* L.) Kuntze "Canary Island Broom"
Fabaceae
Canary Islands. Naturalized in California, Mexico
Rocky hillsides, dry places, heaths, etc.
An evergreen, much-branched shrub to 2 m; leaves 3-foliate, small; flowers in many-flowered
  racemes, bright-yellow, petals 12–14 mm long; pod 12–20 mm long, pubescent.
Mild hallucinogen
Cytisine

Datura candida (Pers.) Safford   "Maikoa," "Queen of the Night"
Solanaceae
South America (north)
Forested areas
Shrub or woody tree to 20 m, corolla tube white, 12–15 cm long; foliage oblanceolate, densely
  tomentose; branching dichotomus to sub-dichotomus; fruit a capsule.
Hallucinogen and hypnotic
Scopolamine, hyoscyamine, and atropine

Datura inoxia Mill.   "Toloache"
Solanaceae
Mexico, southwestern United States
Dry open places, disturbed areas
Coarse, scandent annual; leaves ovate, 5–12 cm long; corolla tube white, 15–18 cm long,
  10-toothed; capsules ovoid, 6–6.5 cm in diameter, spiny.
Hallucinogen and hypnotic
Scopolamine, hyoscyamine, and atropine

Datura metel L. (*D. fatuosa* L.)   "Unmata"
Solanaceae
India; naturalized in the Mediterranean region
Waste places, river sands
Pungent, densely hairy, grayish annual to 1.5 m long; leaves entire or shallowly lobed; flowers large, 18–24 cm long, white often flushed with pink; fruit pendulous, spiny.
Hypnotic and hallucinogen
Scopolamine, meteloidine, hyoscyamine, norhyoscyamine, norscopolamine, cuscohygrine, and nicotine

Datura sanguinea R. & P.   "Huanto"
Solanaceae
Peru
Highlands
A tree-like shrub, 1–4 m tall; leaves clustered, narrow-oblong, to 15 cm long; flowers tubular, pendulous, orange-red with yellow nerves; fruit a turbinate capsule, to 6 cm long.
Hallucinogen and hypnotic
Scopolamine, hyoscyamine, and atropine

Datura stramonium L.   "Jimsonweed"
Solanaceae
Cosmopolitan
Waysides, disturbed places, etc.
An erect, few-branched annual; leaves elliptic to ovate, 5–20 cm long; corolla tube white or pale-lavender, 5-toothed, 6–10 cm long; capsules ovoid, 3–5 cm in diameter, spiny or smooth.
Hallucinogen and hypnotic
Scopolamine, hyoscyamine, and atropine

Delphinium consolida L. (*Consolida regalis* S. F. Gray)   "King's Consound"
Ranunculaceae
Most of Europe except the islands and the south, and most of the Balkan peninsula
Fields and dry places
Annual to 50 cm tall; leaf segments all linear; flowers dark or light blue.
Hypnotic
Delphinine, delphinedine, ajacine

Desfontainea spinosa v. *hookeri* (Dun.) Reiche   "Taique," "Chapico"
Desfontaineaceae
Chile
Hillsides or highlands
A shrub, 1.5–2.5 m tall; leaves, holly-like, 5–7 cm long; flowers tubular, red tipped with bright yellow; fruit a yellowish berry.
Hallucinogen
Unidentified

Duboisia myoporoides R. Br.   "Pituri"
Solanaceae
Australia
Forests
A shrub or tree to 12 m; leaves elliptic, 4–8 cm long; flowers white, tiny, bell-shaped, in terminal clusters; fruit a globular black berry.
Stimulant, secondarily a hallucinogen
Scopolamine, hyoscine

Elaeophorbia drupifera (Thonn.) Stapf.   "Kankan," "Dodo"
Euphorbiaceae
Guinea, Sierra Leone
Forests and coastal plains
Tree-like succulent with a milky sap, branching above, to 5 m; branches slightly 5-angled; leaves obovate-elongate, 15–23 cm long; flowers in a cyathium, small.
Hallucinogen (?)
Unidentified principle in the latex

Elaphrium bipinnatum (DC) Schlecht.   "Palo Copal"
Burseraceae
Mexico (south-central)
Dry places
A shrub or sometimes a small tree to 12 m tall; leaves fern-like, with numerous small leaflets; flowers tiny, whitish; fruit a small 3-angled drupe, containing a single seed.
Stuns without impairing motor coordination
Unidentified

Epilobium angustifolium L.   "Fireweed"
Onagraceae
Circumboreal America and Eurasia
Moist soils rich in humus; abundant after fires
Tall perennial to 2 m; leaves numerous, lanceolate; flowers rosy-purple, many in a long, cylindrical, leafless terminal spike; fruit a 4-angled capsule.
Hypnotic used to fortify *Amanita muscaria*
Unidentified

Erythrina sp.   "Coral-Tree"
Fabaceae
Southwestern United States and Mexico, Guatemala
Flat, dry areas
Woody shrubs to fairly large trees, usually spiny; leaves with 3 broad leaflets; flowers usually bright red or scarlet, showy, in dense racemes; fruit a long pod with bright-colored seeds.
Hallucinogenic stupor
Indoles and isoquinolines; imperfectly known erythrinanes

Erythroxylum coca Lam.   "Coca"
Erythroxylaceae
Peru, Bolivia, Ecuador
Highlands
A densely leafy shrub, 1–2 m tall; leaves elliptic, strongly 3-veined, golden-green, 4–7 cm
    long; flowers axillary, white, small; fruit an orange-red drupe.
Euphoriant and stimulant
Cocaine

Foeniculum vulgare Mill.   "Fennel"
Apiaceae
Southern Europe and southwest United States
Waste places, disturbed areas, waysides
A short-lived perennial, 1–2 m tall; leaves 3–4 pinnately compound with the ultimate
    segments thread-like, very aromatic; flowers in large greenish-yellow umbels.
Epileptiform convulsions and hallucinations
Unidentified oil distillate

Galbulimima belgraveana (F. Müll.) Sprague   "Agara"
Himamtandraceae
Papua, New Guinea
Rain forest slopes
A tree to 15 m tall; leaves leathery, 9–14 cm long; branches and undersides of leaves covered
    with peltate scaly indumentum; flowers on short axillary branches, yellowish, many
    stamens; fruit gall-like, turning red with age, to 1 cm in diameter.
Hallucinogen; the narcosis progresses to an ultimate stupor or coma
Himbacine, polycyclic piperidine derivatives

Gelsemium sempervirens L. (Ait.) f.   "Yellow Jessamine"
Loganiaceae
Southeastern United States
Thickets, woodlands, fence rows, and roadsides
Climbing or trailing vine; leaves evergreen, lanceolate to elliptic, 2–70 m long; flowers
    fragrant, bright yellow, usually solitary; fruit a capsule with many seeds.
Hypnotic
Gelsemine, gelseminine, gelsemoidine—all nerve poisons

Gnaphalium polycephalum Michx. (*G. obtusifolium* L.)   "Sinjachu"
Asteraceae
Most of the eastern United States and Canada, south to Texas
Open sandy places
Annual or maybe biennial, fragrant herb to 1 m tall; leaves numerous, linear-lanceolate, green
    above, white woolly below; flowers in a many-branched, flat or round-topped, often
    elongate inflorescence.
Hypnotic
Unidentified

Gomortega keule Johnston   "Keule," "Hualhual"
Gomortegaceae
Chile
Forest slopes
A large tree to 25 m; leaves aromatic, evergreen shiny; flowers in axillary and terminal
    racemes or panicles; fruit drupaceous with a bony endocarp, 2–3 seeded.
Hallucinogen or, possibly, irritant
Essential oils in the fruit

Gymnopilus spectabilis (Fr.) A. H. Smith (*Pholiota spectabilis* Fr.)
    "Waraitake," "Maitake"
Agaricaceae
Widely distributed in the United States; also Japan
Earth, buried wood, stumps and logs of hardwoods and conifers
Pileus convex, nearly flat in age, dry, buff, yellow to yellow-orange, hairless or hairy in age;
    spores orange or rusty-orange; lamellae adnate to short decurrent, crowded, mustard-
    yellow to orange-buff; stipe to 20 cm long, same color as pileus above, sometimes
    club-shaped; veil membranous, persistent.
Hallucinogen
Unknown

Heimia salicifolia (HBK) Link & Otto   "Sinicuichi"
Lythraceae
Texas, Mexico, and Central America
Along streams
A spreading, branched shrub to 3 m; leaves linear-lanceolate, 2–5 cm long; flowers yellow,
    petals early deciduous; fruit an obovoid ribbed capsule.
Hallucinations, primarily auditory; vision suffused with yellow
Sinicuichine, cryogenine

Homalomena ereriba Schott.
Araceae
Papua, New Guinea
Rain forest slopes
Terrestrial herb from short rootstock; leaves dark-green above, paler beneath; spathe
    greenish.
Questionable, admixture to *Galbulimima belgraveana*
Unidentified

Humulus lupulus L.   "Hop"
Cannabaceae
Europe, Asia, North America
Hedges, damp places, cultivated
Climbing perennial vine; leaves oval, 3–5 lobed, toothed, 10–15 cm long; flowers dioecious,
    male inflorescences branched, pendulous, female stalked, cone-like; fruit an achene in
    cone-like clusters
Sedating, soporific
Unidentified principles in the resins

Hyoscyamus niger L.   "Henbane"
Solanaceae
Europe
Waste places, waysides, sandy areas
A coarse, sticky, hairy biennial or annual, 20–80 cm tall; leaves oblong, 15–20 cm; flowers
    dull-yellow with a network of purple veins; fruit a capsule enclosed by the papery calyx.
Hallucinogen and sedative
Hyoscyamine and scopolamine

Ilex cassine L.   "Dahoon," "Black Drink"
Aquifoliaceae
Southeastern United States
Cypress ponds and bogs
Large shrub or small tree; leaves elliptic to lanceolate, coriaceous, 28 cm long; staminate
    flowers in short, axillary compound cymes; pistillate flowers solitary or in 3-flowered
    cymes; fruit drupaceous, bright red.
Hypnotic
Unknown

Ilex paraguayensis St. Hil.   "Maté"
Aquifoliaceae
Brazil, Argentina, Paraguay
Near streams
An evergreen shrub or small tree to 7 m; leaves serrate, elliptic-obovate, 2.5–8 cm long;
    flowers tiny, white, in axillary clusters; fruit a reddish berry.
Stimulant
Caffeine

Iochroma fuschioides (H. B. K. Miers)   "Borrachero"
Solanaceae
Andean area of Ecuador
Forests
Large shrub to 2 m or more; leaves glabrous, ovate, 5–12 cm long; flowers orange-scarlet,
    tubular, 5 cm long.
Hallucinations
Unidentified

Ipomoea violacea L. (*Ipomoea rubro-coerulea* Cav.)   "Quiebra Plata"
Convolvulaceae
Mexico
Hillsides, most thickets, etc.
A twining vine; leaves cordate-ovate, to 7 cm long and nearly as wide; corolla funnelform,
    violet-blue to reddish-purple; fruit a several-seeded capsule.
Hallucinogen
Amides of lysergic acid

Justicia pectoralis Jaq. v. *stenophylla* Leonard   "Bolek-hena"
Acanthaceae
Venezuela, northern Brazil
Forests
An erect herb to 20 cm tall; leaves narrowly lanceolate; 2–6 cm long; flowers purple, white, or
   lilac, in elongate, mostly one-sided spikes; fruit capsular.
Hallucinogen
Tryptamines (?)

Kaempferia galanga L.   "Maraba"
Zingiberaceae
New Guinea
Usually in open grassy areas
A smooth stemless herb arising from a tuberous aromatic rootstock; leaves orbicular,
   spreading horizontally, 7–15 cm long; flowers white or pale-pink with violet spot
   prominent.
Hallucinogen
Unidentified principle in volatile oils of the rhizome

Lactuca quercina L.   "Wild Lettuce"
Asteraceae
Central and eastern Europe from Bulgaria north to central Germany and south-coast Russia
Woods and scrubland
Erect annual or biennial to 1.5 m tall with thin leaves, sagittate-amplexicaul base; flowers
   yellow in a dense corymbose panicle.
Hypnotic
Lactucarium

Lactuca virosa L.   "Wild Lettuce"
Asteraceae
Central and southern Europe
Waysides, uncultivated ground, rocky places
Stiff, erect biennial to 1.5 m tall with the blades of the stem leaves held horizontally; leaves
   lobed or toothed, sometimes entire; flowers yellow in a lax, much-branched leafless
   inflorescence.
Hypnotic
"Lactucarium," an imperfectly characterized complex from the laticifers of the plant.

Lagochilus inebrians Bunge.   "Intoxicating Mint"
Lamiaceae
Central Asia, Russia
Steppes
A shrub to 1 m tall, leaves 3-lobed, each lobe spine-tipped, pubescent; 1.5–2.5 cm long; calyx
   spiny, ribbed; corolla white, covered with silvery hairs; fruit a nutlet.
Tranquilizer (hallucinogen ?)
Lagochiline and/or a polyhydric alcohol

Latua pubiflora (Gris.) Phil.   "Latue"
Solanaceae
Chile
Moist shaded areas
A spiny shrub or small tree, 3 m or more high; leaves lanceolate, 4–6 cm long; flowers violet,
    axillary; fruit a lemon-yellow berry.
Hallucinogen
Atropine and scopolamine

Leonorus sibricus L.   "Siberian Motherworth," "Marahuanilla"
Lamiaceae
Endemic to Siberia and China; naturalized in the eastern United States, tropical America, and
    the Gulf Coast
Waste places
Biennial with stems to 1.5 m tall; leaves broadly ovate to rotund in outline, deeply 3-parted,
    laciniately toothed; flowers in axillary whorls subtended by bracteal leaves and linear
    bracts, pink; plant strong-scented.
Euphoriant and hypnotic
Leonurine

Leonotis leonurus R. Br. "Lion's Ear," "Lion's Tail," "Dagga," "Twalainoyani"
Lamiaceae
South Africa
Grassland
Branched shrubby perennial, 1–2 m tall, leaves lanceolate, 4–12 cm long, serrate; flowers in
    dense axillary whorls, bright orange-red, pubescent; fruit consisting of four nutlets.
Mild euphoriant
Unidentified resins from the inflorescence

Lobelia tupa L.   "Tupa," "Tabaco del Diablo"
Lobeliaceae
Chile
Wooded slopes, in open and among shrubs
A stately perennial herb, 1.5–2.5 m tall; leaves lanceolate, 16–20 cm long; flowers bright
    scarlet-red, in long terminal racemes; fruit a capsule.
Hallucinogenic stupor
Lobeline and its keto- and dihydroxy derivatives

Lophophora williamsii (Lem.) Coult.   "Peyote," "Mescal Button"
Cactaceae
Texas, north Mexico
Deserts
A small, globose cactus with a carrot-shaped taproot, c. 4 cm high and 6–10 cm in diameter;
    surface blue-green; flowers small, pale-pink or white.
Hallucinogen
Mescaline and over thirty phenylethylamines and simple isoquinolines

Lycoperdon marginatum Heim   "Gi'-i-sa-wa"
Lycoperdaceae
Oaxaca, south, around San Miguel (Mixtec)
Above 2000 m in mountain meadows
"Puffball" with a membranous peridium and a dense white interior when immature; at
    maturity the interior darkens and crumbles to a dark mass of spores; opening by apical
    perforations.
Hallucinogen
Unidentified alkaloid in mature spores (psilocybine (?), Ibotenic acid (?)

Lycopodium selago L.   "Fir Clubmoss"
Lycopodiaceae
With its varieties, circumpolar
Woods, bogs and heaths
Stems short, ascending and divided regularly into branches of equal length; leaves imbricate,
    in many rows along the stem.
Hypnotic
Lycopodine (?)

Mandragora officinarum L.   "Mandrake," "Mandragora," "Satan's Apple"
Solanaceae
Southern Europe
Stony places, deserted cultivation
A perennial with a stout, often branched taproot to 1 m long; leaves in a basal rosette, to 25
    cm long; flowers violet, bell-shaped, on a short stalk, 2–5 cm high; fruit a round, smooth,
    deep-yellow berry.
Hallucinogen; followed by a death-like somnolence
Scopolamine, hyoscyamine, mandragorine, and atropine

Methysticodendron amesianum Schultes   "Culebra-Borrachera"
Solanaceae
Southern Colombia
Forested mountain areas
A tree to 5 m; leaves long-linear, crenulate, 12–25 cm or more; flowers long-tubular, to 25 cm
    or more; white.
Hallucinogen
Hyoscyamine, norhyoscyamine and scopolamine

Mimosa hostilis Benth.   "Vino de Jurema"
Mimosaceae
Brazil
Forests
A viscid puberulent shrub; leaves compound pinnate; flower's spikes c. 2.5–5 cm long;
    corolla 4-parted, 8 stamens; legume viscid puberulent, flat.
Hallucinogen
Unidentified

Mirabilis multiflora (Torr.) Gray   "So'ksi"
Nyctaginaceae
Arizona, Utah, New Mexico, Texas and northern Mexico
On hillsides and mesas, often among rocks and shrubs
An herbaceous perennial, somewhat scandent; leaves ovate, to 4 cm long; corolla tube often
     exceeding 4.5 cm, purple-red, generally more than 3 flowers in each involucre; fruit a
     ribbed achene.
Hallucinogen (?)
Unidentified

Mitchella repens L.   "Partridge Berry"
Rubiaceae
Eastern United States, Canada, Mexico, and Japan
Dry or moist woods
Trailing perennial, forming mats; stems rooting at the nodes; leaves evergreen, round-ovate,
     less than 2 cm long; flowers in pairs, mostly terminal, small, white or tinged pink; berry
     red.
Hypnotic
Unidentified

Mitragyna speciosa Korth.   "Kutum," "Kratom," "Mambog"
Rubiaceae
Malay peninsula
Open country
A large tree, 12–16 m tall; leaves oblong-ovate, 8–12 cm long; flowers in globose heads of 3,
     deep-yellow; seeds winged.
Hallucinogen
Mitragynine and eight similar compounds

Monadenium lugardae N. E. Br.   "Tshulu," "Mhlebe"
Euphorbiaceae
South Africa
Arid plains; open places
Fleshy succulent with a tuberous root, 12–60 cm high; leaves terminally crowned, spatulate,
     1.5–9 cm long; flowers in solitary cymes, greenish; fruit a 3-angled capsule.
Hallucinogen
Methylamines (uncertain)

Monotropa uniflora L.   "Corpse Plant," "Indian Pipe"
Monotropaceae
Most of the United States and Canada south to Central America
Rich woods in leaf-mold
Saprophytic plant lacking chlorophyll, to 25 cm tall; leaves reduced to scales; flowers
     urceolate, white, nodding and solitary.
Hypnotic
Undetermined

Myristica fragrans Houtt.   "Nutmeg"
Myristicaceae
Moluccas, Banda Islands, Malayan archipelago
Open areas of the tropics
A tree to 8 m tall; leaves elliptic, 8–12 cm long; flowers dioecious, small; fruit a pendulous
    globose drupe, splitting into 2 valves disclosing the scarlet aril or mace surrounding the
    seed which is encased in a hard shell.
Hallucinogen
The oils myristicin and elemecin (a fraction of the former)

Nanathus albinotus (Haw.) Bol. [*Rabiea albinota* (Haw.) Br.] "S'Keng-keng"
Aizoaceae
South Africa
Dry open places
Dwarf, compact succulent; leaves fleshy, sabre-shaped, 3-angled above, covered with whitish
    flecky prominent dots; flowers yellowish.
Hallucinogen
Unidentified

Nicotiana rustica L.   "Turkish Tobacco"
Solanaceae
Eastern United States
Waste places, open areas, etc.
A strong-smelling, glandular, hairy annual, 30–100 cm tall; leaves stalked, ovate-cordate,
    6–10 cm long; flowers in dense terminal clusters, greenish-yellow; fruit a many-seeded
    capsule.
Protoplasmic poison and retardant to neural transmission
Nicotine primarily, harman

Nicotiana tabacum L.   "Tobacco"
Solanaceae
Of hybrid and tetraploid origin. Brazilian progenitors
Cultivated
An erect, acrid annual, 1–2 m tall; leaves clasping, ovate-lanceolate, 20–45 cm long; flowers
    pale-pink or purple, in terminal clusters; fruit a many-seeded capsule.
Protoplasmic poison and retardant to neural transmission
Nicotine primarily, harman

Nymphaea ampla (Salisb.) D. C.   "Quetzalaxochiatl," "Precious Water-lily,"
"White Water-lily"
Nymphaeaceae
Tropical and subtropical America from Mexico to Brazil
Aquatic perennial with submerged rootstocks and floating leaves
Leaves sub-orbicular, to 4 cm across, with sinuate margins; flowers white, 12 cm in diameter,
    with 7 to 21 petals.
Hypnotic and hallucinogen
Aporphine (an apomorphine-like alkaloid), nupharine, nupharidine

Nymphaea caerulea Sav.   "Sacred Lily of the Nile," "Blue Water-lily"
Nymphaeaceae
Northern and central Africa
Aquatic perennial with submerged rootstocks and floating leaves
Leaves sub-orbicular, 1–1.5 m in diameter, with more or less entire margins, purple-spotted
    beneath; flowers 9–18 cm in diameter, pale blue with a white center open only in the
    forenoon for 3 days.
Hypnotic and hallucinogen
Nupharine, nuciferine, nupharidine and possibly aporphine

Olmedioperebea sclerophylla Ducke   "Rape dos Indios"
Moraceae
Brazil
Rain forests
A large tree, 25–35 m tall; leaves ovate, 20–30 cm long; male and female flowers borne in
    separate receptacles, small; fruit a drupe, 2–2.5 cm in diameter.
Hallucinogen
Undetermined

Pancratium trianthum Herb.   "Kwashi"
Amaryllidaceae
West Africa
Open places
Perennial arising from a globose-ovoid bulb; leaves linear, flaccid, elongate; flowers whitish
    with a broad pink band up the outer lobes, the tube 12–15 cm long.
Hallucinogen
Unidentified

Paneolus papilionaceus Fr.   "Waraitake," "Maitake"
Agaricaceae
Eastern United States and Canada, Japan
Soil and rich dung
Pileus somewhat fleshy, at first hemispherical, sometimes subumbonate, the cuticle
    breaking up into scales when dry, pale-gray with a tinge of reddish-yellow, c. 2.5 cm
    broad; lamellae broadly attached to the stipe, black; stipe to 10 cm long, slender, firm,
    hollow, whitish, sometimes with red or yellow tinge.
Hallucinogen
Probably psilocybin and psilocin, both of which are present in *Paneolus sphinctrinus*

Passiflora incarnata L.   "Coanenepilli," "Serpent's Tongue"
Passifloraceae
Southeast United States
Fields, roadsides, fence rows, and thickets

Trailing or climbing vine to 2 m long; leaves palmately 3-lobed; flowers axillary, solitary, bluish-white, the corona segments lavender-white, banded with purple; fruit a green or yellow berry to 7 cm long.
Euphoriant and hypnotic
Passicol, harmol, harman, harmine, harmalol, and harmaline

Passiflora jorullensis H.B.K.   "Coanenepilli"
Passifloraceae
Mountains of central and southern Mexico
Forests
Trailing or climbing vine; leaves bilobed or trilobed one-third of their length, the lobes rounded or subacute, mucronulate, 6 cm long; flowers in axillary pairs, orange-red, small; fruit globose, 5 cm in diameter, lustrous black.
Euphoria similar to *Cannabis*
Passicol, harmol, harman, harmine, harmalol, and harmaline

Papaver somniferum L.   "Opium Poppy"
Papaveraceae
Central Europe, the Levant
Fields, waysides, waste places
An erect glaucous annual, 0.5–1.5 m tall; leaves clasping, 7–12 cm long, deeply toothed; flowers to 10 cm across, white, lilac, or purple with or without dark basal blotch; fruit a capsule with many seeds.
A feeling of well-being
Morphine, codeine, and twenty-four other alkaloids

Paullinia cupana H.B.K.   "Cupana," "Guarana"
Sapindaceae
Brazil
Forests
A scandent or sub-erect liana; leaves compound, 5-foliate, 10–20 cm long; flowers white, tiny, in panicles; fruit an apiculate capsule, dark red in maturity; seed dark brown.
Stimulant
Caffeine

Peganum harmala L.   "Syrian Rue," "Zit-el-Harmel"
Rutaceae
Turkey, Syria
Waste places, steppes
An erect perennial herb, 30–70 cm tall; leaves finely dissected into linear segments, 3–5 cm long; flowers solitary, white; capsules slightly stalked.
Hallucinogen
Harmine and related indoles

Pernettya furens (H. & A.) Kl.   "Huedhued," "Hierba Loca"
Ericaceae
Chile
Open fields or clearings in woods
A shrub, 1–1.5 m tall; leaves ovate, 2.5–5 cm long, finely serrate; flowers urn-shaped, white, in short nodding racemes; fruit a many-seeded berry enclosed by the persisting calyx.
Hallucinogen
Possibly andromedotoxine and/or arbutin

Pholiota spectabilis Fr. *(Gymnopilus spectabilis)*   "Waraitake," "Maitake"
Agaricaceae
Southern Canada, mountains of western United States, central and eastern states, Japan
Decayed oak stumps
Stipe, 7–10 cm tall, thick, tough, spongy and thickened toward the base; pileus, compact, convex, then plane, dry, torn into silky scales which disappear toward the margin, golden-orange in color; gills, narrow, crowded, yellow then ferruginous.
Hallucinogen
Unidentified

Phytolacca americana L.   "Pokeweed"
Phytolaccaceae
Much of the eastern United States
Waste ground and pastures, usually disturbed habitats
Robust perennial to 2 m tall with one to many stems from the root crown; roots thick and fleshy; leaves lanceolate, entire, 4–11 cm long; flowers racemose, green to whitish; berry purplish-black at maturity.
Hypnotic, may induce respiratory failure
Phytolacine

Piper betel L.   "Betel"
Piperaceae
Southeast Asia, Polynesia
Shaded wooded areas
A glabrous climbing vine; leaves fleshy, ovate, 10–14 cm long; male spikes cylindric, female spikes to 4 cm long; fruit a drupe.
Unknown (additive to *Areca*)
Unidentified

Piper methysticum Forst.   "Kava Kava"
Piperaceae
Polynesia, Sandwich Islands, South Sea Islands
West forests
A shrub, 1.5–4 m tall; leaves cordate-ovate, 13–22 cm long and almost as wide; flowers dioecious in densely flowered short spikes.
A state of well-being followed by somnolence
Marindin, dihydromethylsticin, and others

Psilocybe sp.   "Magic Mushroom"
Agaricaceae
Narcotic sp. (Sect. Caerulescentes) Mexico and Central America
Sticks, stems, mud, peat, earth, humus, deep moss beds, dung, sawdust, straw, or dead wood
Pileus cylindric conic or semiglobate to convex, campanulate, often umbonate or papillate,
    viscid or dry; spores deep lilac to sepia; stipe not viscid, glabrous or with a fibrillose
    coating; lamellae broad, adnexed to adnate; a few species annulate.
Hallucinogen
Psilocybin and psilocin

Psychotria viridis R. & P.
Rubiaceae
Ecuador, Peru
Forests, western Amazon
A shrub or small tree to 4.5 m tall; leaves obovate or ovate-oblong, 6–9 cm long; inflorescence
    spicate-paniculate, many flowered; flowers whitish, minute; fruit baccate, red.
Hallucinogen
N,N-dimethyltryptamine

Rauvolfia tetraphylla L. (*Rauvolfia canescens* L.)   "Pinque-pinque"
Apocynaceae
Central and northern South America, West Indies
Savannahs
Shrub to 1 m tall; leaves usually in whorls of four, the members of a whorl unequal, ovate,
    4–12 cm long; flowers in axillary and terminal cymes, greenish-white, tiny; fruit a red
    drupe, becoming black.
Tranquilizer
Reserpine (?)

Rauvolfia serpentina (L.) Bth.   "Sarpaganda"
Apocynaceae
India, Malaysia
Sunny or shaded, periodically dry localities
Shrub to 1 m tall; leaves oblong or elliptic, 7–25 cm, usually 3-verticillate; flowers in cymes,
    corolla tube slender, reddish-pink; fruit a globose black drupelet.
Tranquilizer
Reserpine

Rhyncosia longiracemosa Mart. & Gal.   "Piule"
Fabaceae
Southern Mexico
Moist wet thickets or forest, often on limestone
An herbaceous vine, varying in size; leaves 3-foliate, leaflets, 4–7 cm long; flowers in long
    many-flowered racemes; corolla wings yellow, standard reddish-brown; pod contains
    small, compressed dark-brown seeds.
Hallucinogen
Cystine

Rhyncosia pyramidalis (Lam.) Urban   "Piule"
Fabaceae
Southern Mexico, Guatemala
In wet to dry thickets
An herbaceous vine, varying in size; leaves 3-foliate leaflets, 3–12 cm long; flowers in
    racemes; corolla reddish-yellow; pod contains scarlet seeds with a black end.
Hallucinogen
Cystine

Rivea corymbosa Hall. [*Turbina corymbosa* (L.) Raf.]   "Ololiuqui"
Convolvulaceae
Mexico
Moist or wet thickets, often weedy in hedges
A large to small woody vine, often climbing over small trees; leaves ovate-cordate, 4–10 cm
    long; flowers funnelform, white, in dense panicles; fruit a 1-seeded capsule.
Hallucinogen
Ergine, isoergine and minor alkaloids

Salvia divinorum Epl. & Jativa   "Pipiltzintzintli"
Lamiaceae
Mexico
Moist places in ravines
A perennial sprawling herb, to 3 m or more; leaves ovate, 12–15 cm long; flowers white,
    subtended by violet bracts, verticillate on an inflorescence 30–40 cm long; fruit a nutlet.
    Originally described by Epling as having blue flowers.
Hallucinogen
Unidentified (in study by Sandoz Laboratories)

Sarcostemma acidum Voight (*Sarcostemma brevistigma* W. & A.)   "Soma"
Asclepiadaceae
India
Stony places
A twining, leafless sub-shrub; branches cylindrical; flowers in umbels terminating short
    lateral branches, greenish-white; fruit a bivalved follicle; seeds comose.
Hallucinations and giddiness
Undetermined

Sceletium expansum (L.) L. Bol.   "Khana"
Aizoaceae
South Africa
Dry open places
A prostrate shrub to 30 cm high; leaves 4 cm long, lanceolate, persisting after withering as
    skeletons; branches and leaves covered with fine papillae; flowers dull yellow, many
    petals.
Hallucinogen (?)
Mesembrine and mesembrenine

Sclerocarya caffra Sond.   "Marula"
Anacardiaceae
South Africa
Lowveld
A branched tree to 18 m; leaves compound, 7–13 foliate, 15–30 cm long; flowers dioecious, male inflorescences in racemes, female solitary; fruit a yellow, plum-sized drupe.
Hallucinogen (?)
Unidentified

Senecio hartwegii Benth.   "Peyote de Tepic"
Asteraceae
West-central Mexico
Dry places
Shrub; branches, petioles and lower leaf surfaces tomentose; leaves suborbicular; 1–6 cm long, palmately 7–9 nerved, repand-angulate; flower heads yellow, small.
Neurotoxin producing delusions
Pyrrolizidine alkaloids

Solanum nigrum L.   "Black Nightshade"
Solanaceae
Cosmopolitan weed, probably native of Eurasia
Waste places throughout; sometimes in moist ground
Annual, to 1.5 m tall, often widely branched; leaves thin, ovate-lanceolate, acuminate; inflorescences lateral from the internodes, umbelliform, 2–10 flowered; petals white or occasionally pale violet; berries globose black or dark yellow in var. *villosum.*
Neural poison
Solanine

Sophora secundiflora (Ortega) Lag.   "Mescal Bean"
Fabaceae
Texas, New Mexico, and northern Mexico
Usually on limestone hills
Evergreen shrub or occasionally a tree to 9 m; compound leaves deep-green, 8–14 cm long; flowers in pendulous racemes, mauve-violet, very fragrant; pod to 10 cm long containing 1–8 red seeds.
Hallucinogen (highly toxic)
Cystine (ulexine, baptitoxine, sophorine)

Stipa vaseyi Scribn. [*S. robusta* (Vasey) Scribn.]
"Popoton Sacaton," "Sleepy grass"
Poaceae
Colorado to western Texas, Arizona, and northwestern Mexico
Dry plains and hills and dry open woods
Perennial grass to 1–1.5 m tall; panicle compact, larger than in *S. viridula,* plants robust; glumes firm with inconspicuous nerves.
Hypnotic
Unidentified

Stipa viridula Trin.   "Green Needlegrass"
Poaceae
Central Canada, central and eastern United States, southwest to Arizona
Plains and dry slopes
Perennial grass to 1 m tall; panicle slender and loose, plants rather slender; glumes thin and
     papery.
Hypnotic
Unidentified

Stropharia sp.   "Magic Mushroom"
Agaricaceae
Narcotic species in western United States, Mexico, Central and South America, Hawaii, etc.
Soil, foliage, dung; rarely on decayed wood or sawdust
Pileus viscid or humid, white or bright colored; spores deep lilac to blackish lilac (when
     fresh); stipe straight or somewhat flexous, longer than the diameter of the pileus, always
     annulate; lamellae (gills) adnexed to adnate; veil usually membranous.
Hallucinogen
Psilocybin and psilocin

Tagetes lucida Car.   "Yauhtli," "Hierba de Nube"
Asteraceae
Mexico
Woods, hillsides, rocky slopes
Perennial aromatic herb, to 1 m tall; leaves lanceolate, finely serrate; flowers bright yellow in
     dense terminal cymes.
Benumbing (classic náhuatl use), confusion
Coumarins, lactones, and terpenes

Tabernanthe iboga Baill.   "Iboga"
Apocynaceae
Gabon and parts of the Congo
Forests
Shrub 1–2 m tall; leaves lanceolate; opposite, to 14 cm long; inflorescence subumbellate;
     flowers white spotted pink, contorted in bud; fruit a berry; seeds with fleshy ruminate
     albumen; root yellowish.
Hallucinogen
Ibogaine

Tetrapteris methystica Schultes   "Caapi-pinima"
Malpighiaceae
Brazil
Rain forest
A liana; leaves obovate to oblong, 1–3 cm long, light-green above, ash-grey beneath; flowers
     yellow with reddish markings; fruit a samara.
Hallucinogen
Imperfectly known; probably beta-carbolines

Thea sinensis L. (*Camellia sinensis* Kuntze)   "Tea," "Cha"
Theaceae
China, India
Shaded areas
A shrub or occasionally a tree to 10 m; leaves elliptic, 4–10 cm long, leathery; flowers white, usually solitary; fruit a woody capsule.
Stimulant
Theine (caffeine)

Theobroma cacao L.   "Cacao"
Sterculiaceae
Central and South America
Forests of high humidity
A wide-branching tree to 9 m; leaves oblong-oval or elliptic-oblong, to 25 cm long; flowers in fascicles on bark of trunk and main branches, small, yellowish; fruit a woody drupe with numerous seeds.
Stimulant
Theobromine (caffeine)

Trichocereus pachanoi Brit. & Rose   "San Pedro"
Cactaceae
Ecuador
Mountain slopes
A tall columnar cactus, 3–6 m high, with numerous branches; flowers large, white, 19–23 cm long, borne near the tops of the branches, night-blooming, fragrant.
Hallucinogen
Mescaline primarily

Vaccinium uliginosum L.   "Bog Bilberry"
Ericaceae
Circumboreal America and Eurasia
Bogs
Low, dense, much-branched undershrub to .75 m tall; leaves deciduous, elliptic, 3–7 cm long; flowers pink, in clusters of 1–4 from the axils of bud-scales; fruit dark blue or black.
Hypnotic
Unidentified neural toxin

Valeriana officinalis L.   "Valerian"
Valerianaceae
Throughout Europe; naturalized in the United States
Damp places, wet meadows, woods, watersides
Robust perennial herb to 2 m tall; leaves compound, leaflets variable; flowers in dense, terminal, flat-topped, branched clusters, pale pink; stamens 3; fruit crowned with a pappus.
Hypnotic
Monoterpene valepotriotes

Vanda roxburghii R. Por. (syn. *V. tessellata*)   "Tesselated Vanda"
Orchidaceae
Ceylon, India, and Burma
Epiphytic herb of wet forest
Stem, 80 cm tall; densely leafy; inflorescence suberect or ascending; flowers to 5 cm in diameter, usually with green petals and sepals mottled with brown, lip 3-lobed, violet purple.
Hypnotic; delirium and trance states
Unidentified

Veratrum album L.   "White False Helleborine"
Liliaceae
Throughout most of Europe, except Great Britain
In hills and mountains, in pastures and damp grassy places
Robust, erect perennial to 1.5 m tall; leaves numerous, hairy beneath, strongly veined, in whorls of 3; inflorescence a large, branched, elongated terminal cluster; flowers white within, greenish outside, c. 5 cm across, spreading like a star.
Hypnotic
Veratrine and protoveratrine A & B

Virola calophylla Warb.   "Epena," "Parica," "Yakee"
Myristicaceae
Colombia, Brazil
Rain forest
A tree to 20 m, dioecious; leaves leathery, oblong, 20–50 cm long, puberulent beneath; branches and inflorescence also puberulent; flowers in fascicles, small; fruit ellipsoid.
Hallucinogen
N,N-dimethyltryptamine and 5-methoxy-N,N-dimethyltryptamine

Withania somnifera (L.) Dunal   "Ashwagandha," "Kuthmithi"
Solanaceae
South Africa, tropical Africa, India
Open places, disturbed areas, etc.
A much-branched shrub to 2.5 m tall; leaves elliptic to ovate-lanceolate, 6–9 cm long; flowers in axillary fascicles, small, green; fruit a red berry enclosed by the inflated calyx.
Sedative and tranquilizer
Somniferine

A Bibliography of Primary Sources

For reason of limitation of space, works of primary importance and works with thorough bibliographies are represented here. A bibliography of any merit on narcotic plants would necessarily run to several volumes.

Aaronson, B., and H. Osmond. *Psychedelics: The Use and Implications of Hallucinogenic Drugs.* Garden City, N.Y.: Doubleday, 1970.

Aberle, D. *The Peyote Religion Among the Navaho.* Chicago: Aldine, 1966.

Allegro, J. M. *The Sacred Mushroom and the Cross.* Garden City, N.Y.: Doubleday, 1970.

Allen, P. H. "Indians of southeastern Colombia." *Geographical Review* 37 (1947): 580–582.

Altschul, S. von R. *The Genus Anadenanthera in Amerindian Cultures.* Cambridge, Mass.: Harvard Botanical Museum, 1972.

Anderson, E. F. "The biogeography, ecology and taxonomy of *Lophophora* (Cactaceae)." *Brittonia* 21 (1969): 299–310.

Andrews, G., and D. Solomon. *The Coca Leaf and Cocaine Papers.* New York and London: Harcourt Brace Jovanovich, 1975.

Barclay, A. S. "New considerations in an old genus: *Datura.*" Harvard University, Cambridge, Mass., *Botanical Museum Leaflets* 18 (1959): 245–272.

Barrau, J. "Nouvelles observations au sujet des plantes hallucinogènes de la Nouvelle-Guinèe." *J. Agric. Trop. Bot. Appl.* 5 (1958): 377–378.

———. "Observations et travaux rècents sur les végétaux hallucinogènes de la Nouvelle-Guinée." *J. Agric. Trop. Bot. Appl.* 9 (1962): 245–249.

Borheggyi, S. A. "Miniature mushroom stones from Guatemala." *Am. Ant.* 26 (1961): 498–504.

Bravo, H. *Las Cactaceas de Mexico.* Instituto de Biologia, Universidad Nacional de Mexico, 1937.

———. "Una revisión del género *Lophophora.*" *Cact. Succ. Mex.* 12 (1967): 8–17.

Bristol, M. L. "Notes on the species of tree daturas." Harvard University, Cambridge, Mass., *Bot. Mus. Leafl.* 21 (1966): 229–248.

———. "Tree *Datura* drugs of the Colombian Sibundoy." Harvard University, Cambridge, Mass., *Bot. Mus. Leafl.* 22 (1969): 165–227.

Brough, J. "Soma and *Amanita muscaria.*" *Bulletin of the School of Oriental and African Studies* 34 (1971): 331–362.

Campbell, T. N. "Origin of the Mescal Bean Cult." *American Anthropologist* 60 (1958): 156–160.

Castaneda, C. *The Teachings of Don Juan, A Yaqui Way of Knowledge.* Berkeley and Los Angeles: University of California Press, 1968.

Clark, W. G., and J. Del Giudice. *Principles of Psychopharmacology.* New York and London: Academic Press, 1970.

Cooper, J. M. "Stimulants and narcotics. *Handbook of South American Indians.*" U.S. Govt. Printing Office, Washington, D.C., *Bur. Am. Ethnol. Bull.* 143 (1949): 525–558.

Der Marderosian, A. H. "The distribution of indole alkaloids among certain species and varieties of *Ipomoea, Rivea,* and *Convovulus* (Convovulaceae)." *Lloydia* 29 (1966): 35–42.

DeRopp, R. S. *Drugs and the Mind.* New York: Grove Press, 1957.

Diaz, J. L. "Etnofarmacologia de algunos psicotropicos vegetales de Mexico, C.C.C." 4:135–199, Centro Mexicano de Estudios en Farmacodependencia, Mexico, D.F., 1976.

_____. "Ethnopharmacology of sacred psychoactive plants used by the Indians of Mexico." *Ann. Rev. Pharmacol. Toxicol.* 17 (1977): 647–675.

Dobkin de Rios, M. *The Visionary Vine: Psychedelic Healing in the Peruvian Amazon.* New York, Chandler, 1972.

_____. "The influence of psychotropic flora and fauna on Maya religion." *Current Anthropology* 15 (1974): 147–164.

Downing, D. F. "The chemistry of the psychotomimetic substances." *Quart. Rev.* 16 (1962): 133–162.

Efron, D. H. (ed.). *Psychotomimetic Drugs.* New York: Raven Press, 1970.

_____. *Ethnopharmocologic search for psychoactive drugs.* Public Health Serial Publication No. 1645, U.S. Govt. Printing Office, Washington, D.C., 1967.

Emboden, W. A. *Narcotic Plants.* New York: Macmillan, 1972.

_____. "*Cannabis:* a polytypic genus." *Econom. Bot.* 28 (1974): 304–310.

_____. "Dionysus as a shaman and wine as a magical drug." *J. Psy. Drugs* 9 (1977): 187–192.

_____. "The sacred narcotic lily of the Nile: *Nymphaea caerulea.*" *Econom. Bot.,* in press, 1979.

Emboden, W.A., and M. Dobkin de Rios. "*Egyptian and Maya use of the water lily as a narcotic.*" University of Texas Press, 1979.

Emmart, E. W. "Aztec narcotics." *Journ. Am. Pharm. Assn.* 26 (1937): 43–44.

Epling, C., and C. D. Jativa. "A new species of *Salvia* from Mexico." Harvard University, Cambridge, Mass., *Bot. Mus. Leafl.* 20 (1962): 75–76.

Fabing, H. D., and J. R. Hawkins. "Intravenous injection of bufotenine in humans." *Science* 123 (1956): 886–887.

Fadiman, J. "*Genista canariensis:* a minor psychedelic." *Econ. Bot.* 19 (1965): 383–384.

Farnsworth, N. R. "Hallucinogenic plants." *Science* 162 (1968): 1086–1092.

Fernandez, J. W. "*Tabernanthe iboga:* narcotic ecstasis and the work of the ancestors." In Furst (ed.), *Flesh of the Gods: The Ritual Use of Hallucinogens.* New York: Praeger, 1972.

Furst, P. T. *Flesh of the Gods: The Ritual Use of Hallucinogens.* New York: Praeger, 1972.

――――. *Hallucinogens and Culture.* San Francisco: Chandler and Sharp, 1976.

Furst, P. T., and B. G. Myerhoff. "El mito como historia: el ciclo del peyote y la *Datura* entre los huicholes." In *El Peyote y los Huicholes,* edited by S. N. Sitton *et al.,* Setentas No. 29 Mexico, D. F. (1972): 55–108.

Gamage, J. R., and E. Zerkin. *A Comprehensive Guide to the English-Language Literature on Cannabis.* Beloit, Wis.: STASH Press, 1969.

Garner, W. W. *The Production of Tobacco.* Philadelphia, n.p., 1947.

Gatty, R. "Kava—Polynesian beverage shrub." *Econ. Bot.* 10 (1956): 241–249.

Gessner, P. K., and J. H. Page. "Behavioral effects of 5-methy-N,N-dimethyltryptamine, other tryptamines, and LSD." *Am. J. Physiol.* 203 (1962): 167–172.

Giral, F., and S. Ladbaum. "Principio amargo del zacatechichi." *Ciencia* 19 (1959): 243.

Goldsmith, O. *Letters from a Citizen of the World to His Friends in the East,* 2 vols. Bungay, 1820.

Goodman, L. S., and A. Gilman. *The Pharmacological Basis of Therapeutics,* 2nd ed. New York: Macmillan, 1955.

Granier-Doyeux, M. "Native hallucinogenic drugs, Piptadenias." *Bull. Narcotics* 17 (1965): 29–38.

Guzmán, H. G. "Sinopsis de los conocimientos sobre los hongos alucinógenos mexicanos." *Bol. Soc. Bot. Mex.* 24 (1959): 14–34.

Harner, M. J. *The Jivaro: People of the Sacred Waterfall.* New York: Doubleday/Natural History Press, 1972.

――――, ed. *Hallucinogens and Shamanism.* London/New York: Oxford University Press, 1973.

Heim, R. *Les champignons toxiques et hallucinogènes.* Paris: N. Boubée & Cie, 1963.

――――. *Nouvelles Investigations sur les Champignons Hallucinogènes.* Paris: Edit. Mus. Nat. Hist., 1967.

Heim, R., and R. G. Wasson. *Les Champignons Hallucinogènes du Mexique.* Paris: Edit. Mus. Nat. Hist., 1958.

――――. "The mushroom madness of the Kuma." Harvard University, Cambridge, Mass., *Bot. Mus. Leafl.* 21 (1965): 1–36.

Hewitt, R. *Coffee: Its History, Cultivation and Uses.* New York, n.p., 1872.

Hills, K. L. "*Duboisia* in Australia: a new source of Hyoscine and hyoscyamine." *J. of the N. Y. Bot. Gard.* 49 (1948): 185–188.

Hoffer, A., and H. Osmond. *The Hallucinogens.* New York: Academic Press, 1967.

Hofmann, A. "Psychotomimetic drugs. Chemical and pharmacological aspects." *Acta Physiol. Pharmacol. Neerl.* 8 (1959): 240–258.

————. "The discovery of LSD and subsequent investigations on naturally occurring hallucinogens." Chapter 7 in *Discoveries in Biological Psychiatry,* edited by F. Ayd and B. Blackwell (Philadelphia: Lippincott, 1970).

Homstedt, B. "Tryptamine derivatives in epené, an intoxicating snuff used by some South American Indian Tribes." *Arch. Int. Pharmacodyn.* 156 (1965): 285–305.

Hough, W. "Kava drinking as practised by the Papuans and Polynesians." *Smithsonian Institution Misc. Coll.* 47 (1904): 85–92.

Howard, J. H. "The mescal bean cult of central and southern plains: an ancestor of the peyote cult?" *Am. Anthrop.* 59 (1967): 75–87.

Hyams, E. *Dionysus, A Social History of the Wine Vine.* New York: Macmillan, 1965.

Hylin, J. W., and D. Watson. "Ergoline alkaloids in tropical wood roses." *Science* 148 (1965): 499–500.

Ingalls, D. H. "Remarks on Mr. Wasson's Soma." *Journal of the American Oriental Society* 91 (1971): 188–191.

Isbell, H. "Comparison of the reactions induced by psilocybin and LSD-25 in man." *Psychopharmacology* 1 (1959): 29–38.

Johnston, T. H., and J. B. Cleland. "History of the aboriginal narcotic pituri." *Oceania* 4 (1933, 1934): 201–223, 269–289.

Joyce, C. R. B., and S. H. Curry, eds. *The Botany and Chemistry of Cannabis.* London: J. & A. Churchill, 1970.

Kabelik, J., and F. Santavy. "*Cannabis* as a medicament." *Bull. Narcotics* 12 (1960): 5–23.

Kaplan, H. R., and M. H. Malone. "A pharmacologic study of nesodine, cryogenine and other alkaloids of *Heimia salicifolia.*" *Lloydia* 29 (1966): 348–359.

Klüver, H. *Mescal and Mechanisms of Hallucinations.* Chicago: University of Chicago Press, 1966.

LaBarre, W. "Old and new world narcotics: a statistical question and an ethnological reply." *Econ. Bot.* 24 (1970): 368–373.

————. *The Peyote Cult.* Rev. and enlarged ed. Hampden, Conn.: Shoestring Press, 1974.

Lewin, L. *Phantastica, Narcotic and Stimulating Drugs, Their Use and Abuse.* London: Kegan Paul, Trench, Trubner, 1931.

Lindesmith, A. R. *Addiction and Opiates.* Chicago: Aldine, 1968.

Linegeman, R.R. *Drugs from A to Z: A Dictionary.* New York: McGraw-Hill, 1969

Lowry, B. "New Records of Mushroom Stones from Guatemala." *Mycologia* 63 (1971): 983–993.

Lumholtz, C. *Unknown Mexico*, vol. 1. New York: Scribners, 1902.

MacDougall, T. "*Ipomoea tricolor:* a hallucinogenic plant of the Zapotecs." *Bol. Centro. Invest. Antrop. Mexico* 6 (1960): 6–8.

Martinez, M. *Las Plantas Medicinales de Mexico*. Ediciones Botas, Mexico, D.F., 1959.

――――. "Las Solandras de Mexico con una specie nueva." *Anales de Instituto de Biologia*, Mexico, D.F., 37 (1 & 2): 97–106, 1966.

McCleary, J. A., P. S. Sypherd, and D. L. Walkington. "Antibiotic activity of an extract of Peyote *Lophophora williamsii* (Lemaire) Coulter." *Econ. Bot.* 14 (1960): 247–249.

Moller, K. O., ed. *Rauschgifte und Genussmittel*. Basel, Switzerland: Benno Schwabe, 1951.

Mortimer, N. G. *History of Coca, the Divine Plant of the Incas*. San Francisco: Fitz Hugh Ludlow Memorial Library reprint of the New York 1901 ed. and/or Press, 1974.

Morton, C. V. "Notes on yagé, a drug plant of south-eastern Colombia." *Journ. Wash. Acad. Sci.* 21 (1931): 485–488.

Naranjo, C. *The Healing Journey: New Approaches to Consciousness*. New York: Pantheon Books, 1973.

O'Connel, F. D., and E. V. Lynn. "The alkaloids of *Banisteriopsis inebrians* Morton." *J. Am. Pharm. Assoc.* 42 (1953): 753–754.

Osmund, H. "Ololiuqui: the ancient Aztec narcotic." *Journ. Ment. Sci.* 101 (1955): 526–537.

Pennes, H. H., and P. H. Hoch. "Psychotomimetics, clinical and theoretical considerations: harmine, WIN-2299 and nalline." *Am. J. Psychiatry* 113 (1957): 887–892.

Pinkley, H. V. "Plant admixtures to ayahuasca, the South American hallucinogenic drink." *Lloydia* 32 (1969): 305–314.

Plowman, T., L. Gyllenhaal, and J. Lindgren. "*Latua pubiflora:* magic plant from southern Chile." Harvard University, Cambridge, Mass., *Bot. Mus. Leafl.* 23 (1971): 61–92.

Pollock, S. H. "The Psilocybin Mushroom Pandemic." *Journ. of Psychedelic Drugs* 7 (1975): 73–84.

Pope, H. G. "*Tabernanthe iboga:* an African narcotic plant of social importance." *Econ. Bot.* 23 (1969): 174–184.

Porta, G. B. *Natural Magick*. Reproduction of the 1658 English edition based upon the Italian edition of 1589, New York: Basic Books, 1957.

Prance, G. T. "Notes on the use of plant hallucinogens in Amazonian Brazil." *Econ. Bot.* 24 (1970): 62–68.

Quisumbing, E. *Medicinal Plants of the Philippines*. Manila Bureau of Printing, Technical Bull. 16, 1951.

Ramsbottom, J. *Mushrooms and Toadstools*. London: Collins, 1953.

Reichel-Dolmatoff, G. "Notes on the cultural extent of the use of yajé *(Banisteriopsis caapi)* among the Indians of the Vaupés, Colombia." *Econ. Bot.* 24 (1970): 32–33.

Ristic, S., and A. Thomas. "Zur Kentniss von *Rhynchosia pyramidalis* (Pega-Palo)." *Arch. Pharmaz.* 295 (1962): 510.

Robichaud, R. C., M. H. Malone, and D. S. Kosersky. "Pharmaco-dynamics of cryogenine, an alkaloid isolated from *Heimia salicifolia* Part II." *Arch. Int. Pharmacodyn. Ther.* 157 (1965): 43–52.

Safford, W. E. "Identity of cohoba, the narcotic snuff of ancient Haiti." *J. Wash. Acad. Sci.* 6 (1916): 548–562.

———. "Narcotic plants and stimulants of the ancient Americans." *Ann. Rep. Smithson. Inst.* 1916 (1917): 387–424.

———. "Synopsis of the genus *Datura*." *J. Wash. Acad.* Sci. 11 (1921): 173–189.

———. "Daturas of the Old World and New: an account of their narcotic properties and their use in oracular and initiatory ceremonies." *Ann. Rep. Smithson. Inst.* 1920 (1922): 537–567.

Sahagún, F. B. de. *The Florentine Codex. General History of the Things of New Spain.* Translated by Arthur J. O. Anderson and Charles E. Dibble. Santa Fe, New Mexico: The School of American Research and the University of Utah, 1950–1963.

Sanford, J. H. "Japan's Laughing Mushrooms." *Econ. Bot.* 26 (1972): 174–181.

Santesson, C. G. "Piule eine mexikanische Rauschdroge." *Ethnol. Stud.* (Gothenburg) 4 (1937): 1–11.

Schleiffer, H. *Sacred Narcotic Plants of the New World Indians: An Anthology of Texts from the Sixteenth Century to Date.* New York: Hafner, 1973.

Schneider, J. A., and E. B. Sigg. "Neuropharmacological studies on ibogaine." *Ann. N. Y. Acad. Sci.* 66 (1957): 765.

Schultes, R. E. "Peyote and plants used in the peyote ceremony." Harvard University, Cambridge, Mass., *Bot. Mus. Leafl.* 5 (1937): 61–88.

———. "Peyote *(Lophophora williamsii)* and plants confused with it." Harvard University, Cambridge, Mass., *Bot. Mus. Leafl.* 5 (1937): 61–88.

———. "Plantae Mexicanae II. The identification of teonanacatl, a narcotic Basidiomycete of the Aztecs." Harvard University, Cambridge, Mass., *Bot. Mus. Leafl.* 7 (1939): 37–54.

———. "A contribution to our knowledge of *Rivea corymbosa*, the narcotic oloiuqui of the Aztecs." Cambridge, Mass.: Harvard Botanical Museum, 1941.

———. "A new narcotic snuff from the northwest Amazon." Harvard University, Cambridge, Mass., *Bot. Mus. Leafl.* 16 (1954): 241–260.

———. "The identity of the malpighiaceous narcotics of South America." Harvard University, Cambridge, Mass., *Bot. Mus. Leafl.* 18 (1957): 1–56.

———. "The search for new natural hallucinogens." *Lloydia,* 29 (1966): 293–308.

———. "The botanical and chemical distribution of hallucinogens." *Ann. Rev. Pl. Physiol.* 21 (1970): 571–594.

Schultes, R. E., and A. Hofmann. *The Botany and Chemistry of Hallucinogens.* Springfield, Ill.: Charles C. Thomas, 1973.

Schultes, R. E., W. M. Klein, T. Plowman, and T. Lockwood. "*Cannabis:* an example of taxonomic neglect." Harvard University, Cambridge, Mass., *Bot. Mus. Leafl.* 23 (1974): 337–360.

Scott, J. *The Mandrake Root.* London, n.p., 1946.

Solomon, D., ed. *The Marihuana Papers.* Indianapolis: Bobbs-Merrill, 1966.

Spruce, R. *Notes of a Botanist on the Amazon and Andes.* Edited by A. R. Wallace. 2 vols. London: Macmillan, 1908.

Steinmetz, E. F. "*Tabernanthe iboga* radix." *Quart. Journ. Crude Drug Res.* I (1961): 30.

Stubbs, H. *The Indian Nectar or a Discourse Concerning Chocolata.* London: Crook, 1662.

Taylor, N. *Plant Drugs That Changed the World.* New York: Dodd, Mead, 1965.

Thevet, A. *Les Singularitez de la France antarcticque . . .* Paris, 1557.

Thompson, C. J. S. *The Mystic Mandrake.* London, New York: University Books, 1968.

Tyler, V. E., Jr. "The physiological properties and chemical constituents of some habit-forming plants." *Lloydia* 29 (1966): 275–292.

Usátegui, N. N. "The present distribution of narcotics and stimulants amongst the Indian tribes of Colombia." Harvard University, Cambridge, Mass., *Bot. Mus. Leafl.* 18 (1959): 273–304.

Usdin, E., and D. H. Efron. *Psychotropic Drugs and Related Compounds.* Pub. Health Serv. Publ. 1589, U.S. Govt. Printing Office, Washington, D.C., 1967.

Wassén, S. H. "Some general viewpoints in the study of native drugs especially from the West Indies and South America." *Ethnos* 1–2 (1964): 97–120.

_____. "The use of some specific kinds of South American Indian snuffs and related paraphernalia." *Etnolog. Stud.* 28 (1965): 1–116.

Wassén, S. H., and B. Homstedt. "The use of paricá, an ethnological and pharmacological review." *Ethnos* 1 (1963): 5–45.

Wasson, R. G. "The divine mushroom: primitive religion and hallucinatory agents." *Proc. Am. Phil. Soc.* 102 (1958): 221–223.

_____. "The hallucinogenic mushrooms of Mexico and psilocybin: a bibliography." Harvard University, Cambridge, Mass., *Bot. Mus. Leafl.* 20 (1962): 25–73.

_____. "A new Mexican psychotropic drug from the Mint Family." Harvard University, Cambridge, Mass., *Bot. Mus. Leafl.* 20 (1962): 25–73.

_____. *Soma, Divine Mushroom of Immortality.* New York: Harcourt Brace Jovanovich, 1967.

Wasson, R. G., C. A. Ruck, and A. Hofmann. *The Road to Eleusis: Unveiling the Secret of the Mysteries.* New York, London: Harcourt Brace Jovanovich, 1978.

Wasson, V. P., and R. G. Wasson. *Mushrooms, Russia and History.* New York: Pantheon, 1957.

Watt, J. M., and M. G. Breyer-Brandwijk. *The Medicinal and Poisonous Plants of Southern and Eastern Africa,* 2nd ed. Edinburgh: Livingstone, 1962.

Weil, A. T. "Nutmeg as a narcotic." *Econ. Bot.* 19 (1965): 194–217.

———. *The Natural Mind.* Boston: Houghton Mifflin, 1972.

Wickizer, V. D. *Coffee, Tea and Cocoa, An Economic and Political Analysis.* Stanford, Cal.: Stanford University Press, 1951.

Wolstenholme, G. E. W., and J. Knight, eds. *Hashish: Its Chemistry and Pharmacology.* Boston: Little, Brown, 1957.

Woodson, R. E., Jr., *et al. Rauwolfia: Botany, Pharmacognosy, Chemistry, and Pharmacology.* Boston: Little, Brown, 1965.

PHOTOGRAPHY CREDITS

I wish to thank the following individuals for permission to allow their photographs to be reproduced in this volume. Numbers correspond to plate numbers.

Robert Gustafson (5,9,12,14,15,16,24,29,31,34,39,40,41,49), Peter Jankay (19,20,21), Helen Kennedy (47), Laurel Woodley (32).

Special thanks are due Armando Solis who worked diligently photographing drawings, paintings and various objects appearing throughout this book.

INDEX

NOTE: *Page numbers in boldface refer to illustrations.*

Porta, Giovanni Battista, 127–28, 129
Portugal, 38, 47, 50
Prance, G. T., 105
Psilocybe, 49, 70, 71; *P. aztecorum*, 89; *P. caerulescens* var. *mazatecorum*, 90; *P. caerulescens* var. *nigripes*, 89–90; *P. cubensis*, 91; *P. mexicana*, 89, 91; *P. semilanceata*, 70; *P. wassonii*, 70; *P. zapotecorum*, 89
psychodysleptics, 1–34
psychotomimetics, *see* hallucinogens
Psychotria nitida, 105; *P. psychotriafolia*, 105; *P. viridis*, **104,** 105
Pterygota alata, 32

Quazilbash, 60

Raleigh, Walter, 37
Rameses III, 11, 156
Rauvolfia, 7–8; *R. serpentina*, 7–8
Ravenel, H. W., 92
Reay, Marie, 69–70, 106
Reichel-Dolmatoff, G., 106
Reko, V. A., 95, 97
Rheum, 59; *R. palmatum*, 59
Rhizopus, 95
rhubarb, 59
Rhynchosia, 83, 88; *R. longiraceomosa*, 88, **89;** *R. pyramidalis* (*R. phaseolides*), 88
Rig-Veda, 58–61, 62–63, 65
Rivea, 68; *R. corymbosa*, 95, **96**
Romans, 29, 151–52, 155, 157
Romero, John, 21–22
Roseocactus (*Ariocarpus*) *fissuratus*, 84
Ross, William, 69
Russula, 70

Saccharomyces cerevisiae, 158
Sacred Mushroom and the Cross, The (Allegro), 65
saffron, 49
sagack-homi, 19–20, 63
Sahagún, F. B. de, 85, 88, 94, 98
Salazar, Cervantes de, 4
Salvia divinorum, 70, 93–95
Sandoz Laboratories, 89, 91, 130
Sanford, James H., 50
Santesson, C. G., 95

Sarcostemma, 60–61, 65; *S. acidum*, 60, 61; *S.* (*Asclepias*) *viminale*, 60; *S. brevistigma*, 59, 60, 61
Sceletium, 75–76; *S. expansum*, 75–76, **75;** *S. tortuosum*, 75–76, **76**
Schlitter, Emil, 7
Schultes, Richard Evans, 45, 89, 95, 101, 105, 106–7, 111, 112, 114, 115, 118, 121
Sclerocarya caffra, 75, **78,** 79
Scythians, 52, **52,** 54, 81
sedatives, 1–34
Sedgwick, Robert, 156
Senecio canicida, 99; *S. hartwegii*, **98,** 99
Shakespeare, William, 1, 2, 11, 44, 46, 154
Sharon, Douglas, 120
Sherley, Anthony, 134
Shu-bad, Queen, 155
Shulgin, Alexander, 46
Siculus, Diodorus, 156
sinicuichi, 83
snake plant, 95
snuffs, 38, 107–15, **108**
Solanaceae family, 95
Solanum, 25, 128; *S. tuberosum*, 154
soma, 52, 58–65
Sonchus oleraceus, 33
Sophora secundiflora, 87–88
South Africa, 75–77
Soviet Union, 9, 154
Spain, 37, 39, 47, 88, 142
Spartium junceum, 34
Spruce, Richard, 37, 101–3, 110–11
Stachys, 100
Stictocardia, 68
stimulants, 132–47
Stipa vaseyi, 18–19, **19;** *S. viridula*, 19
Strombocactus disciformis, 84
Stropharia (*Psilocybe*) *cubensis*, 89, 90

Tabernanthe, 76; *T. iboga*, 71–73, **72**
Tagetes lucida, 98–99
Tastevin, R. P., 107
tea, 132–34, **133**
teonanacatl, 88–91
Tetrapteris methystica, 106–7
teuvetli, 4

Thailand, 32, 49, 132
Thea sinensis, 132, **133**
Theobroma cacao, 137–38, **139;** *T. subincanum*, 112
Theophrastus, I., 10, 54
Thevet, André, 38, 39
Thompson, Charles H., 84
Thomson, Samuel, 21
tobacco, 4, 35–43, 73, 76, 85, 95
tranquilizers, 1–34
Trichocereus pachanoi, 118–21, **119**
Tula tree, 32
Tyler, Varro, 97

United States, 77, 120–21, 131; hypnotics in, 2, 7, 18–19, 23, 31–32; inebriants in, 154, 156, 158; *Pharmacopoeia*, 22, 25; stimulants in, 133, 134, 135, 138, 141; tobacco in, 36, 37, 43

Vaccinium, 20, 62–63, **63**
Valeriana officinalis, 15, **16**
Vanda roxburghii, 17, **17**
Venezuela, 102, 104, 105, 112, 114, 138, 154
Veratrum album, 15, **16**
Vinca major, 8
Vincenzi, Frank, 97
Virola, 110, 111–16; *V. calophylla*, 112, **112;** *V. calophylloidea*, 112; *V. cuspidata*, 111; *V. elongata*, 112, 114; *V. sebifera*, 114; *V. theiodora*, 111, 113, 114
Vitis vinifera, 150–51, 153

Wasson, R. Gordon, 59, 61, 62, 69–71, 89–90, 92, 93, 94, 95, 107
water lilies, 12–13, 26, **90,** 91
Weitlaner, Roberto J., 89
West Indies, 32, 36–37, 79, 100, 111, 140
Whiting, Albert, 82–83
Wilbert, Johannes, 40
wine, 148–53, 155, 156, 159
Withania, 8–9

Yaquis, 34, 97
Yemen, 144, 145

Zapotecs, 95
Zarathustra, 54, 58
Zend-Avesta, 52